Nutritional Disorders of American Women

CURRENT CONCEPTS IN NUTRITION

Myron Winick, Editor

Institute of Human Nutrition
Columbia University College of Physicians and Surgeons

Volume 1: Nutrition and Development
Volume 2: Nutrition and Fetal Development
Volume 3: Childhood Obesity
Volume 4: Nutrition and Aging
Volume 5: Nutritional Disorders of American Women

NUTRITIONAL DISORDERS OF AMERICAN WOMEN

Edited by

MYRON WINICK

Institute of Human Nutrition
Columbia University College of Physicians and Surgeons

A WILEY-INTERSCIENCE PUBLICATION

JOHN WILEY & SONS
New York • London • Sydney • Toronto

Library of Congress Cataloging in Publication Data:

Main entry under title:

Nutritional disorders of American women.

(Current concepts in nutrition; v. 5)
Proceedings of a symposium held in New York, Nov. 20–21, 1975.
"A Wiley-Interscience publication."
Includes index.
1. Nutrition disorders—Congresses. 2. Women—Diseases—United States—Congresses. 3. Women—Nutrition—Congresses. I. Winick, Myron. II. Series.
[DNLM: 1. Nutritional disorders—Congresses. 2. Women—Congresses. QZ105 S989n 1975/W1 CU788AS v. 5]
RC620.5.N88 616.3′9 76–54393
ISBN 0–471–02393–0

Printed in the United States of America

10 9 8 7 6 5 4 3 2 1

Preface

This book represents the proceedings of a symposium, Nutritional Disorders of American Women, held in New York City on November 20–21, 1975. The symposium focused on the most serious nutritional problems encountered by women in America. In addition, emphasis was given to those diseases which are more common in women and which have a nutritional component.

The first part of the book explores the special nutritional needs of women as they normally progress through their life cycle. Nutritional needs of pregnancy are examined in experimental animals by Dr. Pedro Rosso, Assistant Professor of Pediatrics in the Institute of Human Nutrition at Columbia University. He discusses animal experiments that have recently challenged the age old concept of the fetus as a "perfect parasite." Outlining a series of experiments by himself and others, Dr. Rosso demonstrates that rat placenta undergoes a progressive maturation during the latter part of pregnancy and that this maturation is essential for normal transport of nutrients from mother to fetus. Maternal malnutrition decreases the capacity of the placenta to transfer glucose and amino acids. In the guinea-pig this has resulted in fetal death and in the rat in fetal growth retardation. The malnourished rat mother actually keeps a higher percentage of nutrients than she normally would. This can be seen if one examines the effect of malnutrition on maternal and fetal body weight. Fetal weight is always proportionally reduced more than maternal weight. Available data suggest that the same is true in humans. Thus the fetus is directly responsive to maternal nutritional status and dependent for proper growth on adequate dietary intake by the mother.

Dr. Roy Pitkin, Professor of Obstetrics and Gynecology at the University of Iowa, extends Dr. Rosso's principles to pregnant women. He notes that the total energy cost of pregnancy, calculated from the amounts of protein and fat accumulated by the mother and fetus, and the additional metabolism incurred by these tissues, amounts to approximately 75,000 kcal. This amounts to an increased requirement of 300 calories per day. The simplest way to assess caloric intake is to monitor weight gain. The usual pattern of gain consists of 1 to 2 kg during the first trimester and then a progressive linear rate of gain averaging 350 to 400 grams per week through the last two-thirds of gestation. Such a course will result in a total gain of 10 to 12 kg. By term the mother has added 2 kg to her blood volume, almost 2 kg to her uterus and breasts, 1 to 2 kg of other fat, and almost 2 kg to her extracellular fluid. In addition, fetus, placenta, and amniotic fluid account for 5 kg directly. Dr. Pitkin goes on to point out that inadequate weight gain during pregnancy may result in fetal growth retardation and that the mother who enters pregnancy already underweight may be at greater risk.

The protein requirement in pregnancy is about 19 g per day more than the nonpregnant requirement and is even greater in the pregnant adolescent. It is estimated that 500 mg of extra iron are utilized by the bone marrow during pregnancy. If one adds the "fetal and placental requirement" (250 to 300 mg), 750 mg of extra iron are needed during the course of a normal pregnancy. This amount is difficult if not impossible to achieve from our ordinary diet and hence routine supplementation is recommended. Folate requirements also increase during pregnancy and if dietary assessment reveals a low intake, then supplements should be given. Requirements for calcium increase to 1200 mg/day and all other minerals and vitamins are required in slightly increased amounts. Dr. Pitkin concludes that the obstetrician must assess the nutritional status of his patient and carefully monitor the patient's diet and weight gain throughout pregnancy.

From pregnancy demands we move to the special nutritional needs of the lactating woman. This subject is covered by Dr. E. M. Widdowson of the Department of Investigative Medicine, University of Cambridge, England. She points out that given the quantity of milk consumed by a normal infant, a lactating mother must take in 600 to 800 kcal above her daily intake. However if she increases her intake by 500 kcal (the increase recommended by the National Research Council) she will consume some of her body stores which have been laid down as fat during pregnancy. Although the efficiency of milk production during lactation is about 90%, extra care should be taken to assure adequate intake of calcium and vitamins A and C.

A relatively new concept introduced by Dr. Widdowson is that some of the tissue changes in the mother that occur during pregnancy are primarily in preparation for lactation The most important of these changes is the deposition of up to 4 kg of fat This is also seen in animals and points up the importance of lactation. Rats at mating contain about 51 g of body fat. By term total body fat was 72 g and after successful lactation for 3 weeks, body fat was 29 g. Thus breast-feeding is an excellent way to lose the fat stored during gestation and if properly monitored might prove a good way to lose excess fat present prior to pregnancy.

Breast milk is amazingly constant in composition. Both marked excess and marked restriction of water intake reduce the quantity of milk. Reduction of calories does the same but the composition, changes very little. This is also true of reduction in protein, carbohydrate or fat. By contrast, the concentration of vitamins and minerals in the maternal diet is reflected in their concentration in breast milk. These first three chapters point up the continuum of gestation and lactation and the importance of nutrition throughout that continuum.

One recent change in the metabolism and in the nutrition of women during the reproductive years has been induced by the widespread use of the contraceptive pill. This subject is discussed by Dr. Daphne Roe, Associate Professor of Nutrition at Cornell University. Certain nutrient requirements appear to be increased by the use of oral contraceptives. These include vitamin B_6, folic acid, and to a lesser extent, riboflavin, thiamine, and ascorbic acid. Clinical evidence of deficiency, although relatively rare, does occur. Vitamin B_6 depletion associated with subjective depression, as well as glossitis from riboflavin deficiency, have been reported. Of most clinical significance are reports of a few cases of megaloblastic anemia secondary to the folic acid deficiency. By contrast plasma levels of certain nutrients increase in women who use the pill, suggesting a possible decrease in the requirement of these nutrients. These include vitamin A, iron, and copper. Dr. Roe concludes that a great deal remains to be learned about the interaction of oral contraceptives and various nutrients. However a diet adequate in those nutrients usually found to be at low levels is recommended. Supplemental vitamins in normal doses might be used but these should not contain vitamin A.

Dr. JoAnne Brasel, Associate Professor of Pediatrics at the Institute of Human Nutrition, Columbia University, discusses nutrient requirements at special periods in the life of the female adolescent. She points out that during this period there is a marked acceleration in growth rate and significant increases in lean body mass, skeletal mass, and adipose tissue. In general, males deposit proportionally more lean body mass and females proportionally more adipose tissue. The implications of these specific tissue changes on nutritional requirements have not been carefully studied. The intense anabolic nature at this time of life increases nutritional requirements and concern is voiced about some of the dietary habits practiced by certain teenagers.

The second part of the book discusses diseases that have a major nutritional component and that have a higher incidence among women. The major diseases considered in detail are anemia, osteoporosis, and obesity. Anemia is discussed by Dr. Victor Herbert, Clinical Professor Pediatrics and Medicine, Columbia University, College of Physicians and Surgeons. The most important anemias in women are iron deficiency anemia and folate deficiency. During the menstrual years women have approximately twice the iron requirements of men. For them, the American diet is marginal in iron, and approximately 40% of women between ages 20 and 50 may have iron depletion. Requirements for folic acid increase with pregnancy and if supplementation is not given, the mother may be depleted. After several pregnancies, the depletion can be compounded if the mother is taking oral contraceptive pills between pregnancies. Dr. Herbert agrees with both the Committee on Maternal Nutrition and the Committee on Dietary Allowances of the Food and Nutrition Board, which recommend that supplementary iron and folate should be given during pregnancy. In addition, he feels that special attention should be paid to these nutrients throughout the reproductive years.

Surveys have shown that a minimum of 10% of the female population over 50 years of age suffer from severe enough osteoporosis to have caused bone loss that potentially could result in hip, vertebrae, or long-bone fractures. Dr. Louis Avioli discusses this problem, pointing out that the overall incidence of osteoporosis in postmenopausal females is approximately 25 to 30%. The cause of this disease has not yet been established. Certainly there is a hormonal component and short-term estrogen therapy immediately after menses may decrease the accelerated rate of bone resorption that occurs at that time. In addition, the relatively low calcium high phosphorus diets in our affluent society may heighten susceptibility to this disease. However, reversal of symptomatic disease by altering calcium-phosphorus ratios in the diet has not proved to be possible. Moreover other therapies such as long-term estrogen administration and supplementation with sodium fluoride have not proved useful according to Dr. Avioli.

Perhaps the most common chronic illness in American women is obesity. Three chapters deal with this subject. Dr. Sami Hashim, Associate Professor of Public Health Nutrition at the Institute of Human Nutrition, Columbia University, discussed appetite control and food intake regulation in man. Using a feeding machine, he shows that lean individuals on a metabolic ward eat a sufficient quantity of food to maintain body weight. Under identical conditions, obese individuals reduce their food intake drastically and lose weight. In addition, when the nutrient content of the dispensed liquid is manipulated, lean individuals adjust the volume of their intake to keep calories consumed constant. Obese individuals are incapable of these adjustments. These data have strengthened the hypothesis that obese individuals regulate their appetite by responding to external environmental clues.

Dr. Mary Greenwood, Assistant Professor of Genetics at the Institute of Human Nutrition, describes some of the newest findings in animals relevant to the differences in obesity rates in males and females. Her studies reveal that in genetically obese rats there is a burst of adipocyte proliferation which occurs at about 14 weeks of age and which does not occur in the lean female rat. If a similar situation is true in the human, then it is possible that childhood obesity might be either more common or more permanent in girls than in boys.

Finally, Dr. Judith Stern, Assistant Professor of Nutrition at the University of California, Davis, attempts to put the data of the previous two chapters into clinical perspective. She demonstrates the uselessness of many of the fad diets and discusses the importance of modifying eating behavior by changing the external cues. In addition, she stresses the importance of preventing obesity, especially in young girls, by regulating caloric intake at an early age, especially in children who demonstrate a tendency toward obesity.

An area much discussed and often abused is the area of vitamins. Dr. Roslyn B. Alfin-Slater, Professor of Nutrition at the University of California at Los Angeles, presents the pros and cons of vitamin supplementation. She acknowledges the fact that vitamin requirements for women change with changes in the life cycle and that especially during pregnancy and lactation, requirements for certain vitamins increase. She deplores, however, the widespread use of vitamin supplements as "insurance policies" in case the daily diet is lacking in these essential nutrients. Moreover the recent proliferation of megavitamin supplements has created a problem with potentially serious repercussions. Dr. Alfin-Slater presents data which indicate that very high doses of vitamin C and E have little therapeutic effect and that toxicity and side effects have been reported with these regimens as well as with excess doses of vitamins A and D.

In the last chapter, Dr Frank W. Lowenstein, examines the most up to date statistics available in this country pertaining to the nutritional status of our female population. The findings emphasize the statistical importance of the issues that were discussed during the symposium. Iron deficiency anemia is a significant problem in all women and particularly among black women during the child-bearing age. Calcium intakes are low and phosphorus intakes high and obesity is extremely prevalent – again more so among black than among white women. Dr. Lowenstein concludes that black women are at highest risk for mortality and morbidity from several major chronic diseases associated with obesity.

MYRON WINICK

New York, New York
February 1977

Contents

Nutritional Disorders of American Women

PART 1

Nutrition and Reproduction

1

Maternal Nutrition, Nutrient Exchange, and Fetal Growth

PEDRO ROSSO, M.D.

Department of Pediatrics, Institute of Human Nutrition, College of Physicians and Surgeons, Columbia University, New York, New York

Most of the phenomena that constitute what is generally termed "maternal-fetal exchange" are directly or indirectly related to two basic characteristics of pregnancy. The first characteristic is the total dependency of the fetus on the maternal supply of nutrients. The second is the incapacity of the mother to support fetal growth throughout gestation, using only her body stores of nutrients, without becoming severely depleted. Such depletion would ultimately reduce the probability of both prenatal and postnatal survival of the young. Thus, the conceptus must induce in the mother certain adaptive changes to ensure an adequate supply of nutrients for itself without depleting the maternal stores. A favorable outcome of pregnancy seems to depend on the ability of the conceptus to elicit such metabolic adaptation of the mother.

The mechanisms modulating the exchange of nutrients between the mother and the fetus are largely unknown. The fact that the fetus derives its sustenance from the mother without making any apparent direct contribution to maternal welfare has fostered the belief that maternal-fetal exchange is basically similar to a host-parasite situation. Furthermore, from this belief has evolved the satellite concept which states that the fetus, because of its parasitic qualities, will thrive even when the mother is moderately malnourished. Data demonstrating that severe degrees of maternal dietary restriction induce only a moderate reduction in birthweight have been interpreted as supporting this idea. However, as we shall discuss later, when the same data are reanalyzed, and the effects of malnutrition on the mother and on the fetus are compared, the results do not unequivocally support the theory that the fetus is a successful parasite. On the contrary, some of the results even suggest that the fetus is proportionally more affected than the mother, hence raising some doubts about the validity of the current ideas on maternal-fetal exchange regulation.

The evidence supporting the possibility that during a period of reduced availability of nutrients the fetus is proportionally more affected than the mother, and our present understanding of maternal-fetal exchange of nutrients during normal pregnancy will be the focus of this chapter.

MATERNAL NUTRITIONAL ADAPTATIONS TO PREGNANCY

Increased food intake and body weight gain are among the earliest visible changes associated with pregnancy in eutherian mammals. In the rat the average daily food intake increases approximately 17 to 20% during pregnancy (1, 2), which represents a cumulative extra intake of approximately 60 g of food. For a standard laboratory diet, containing 25% protein, 65% carbohydrates, and 10% fat, such an intake represents approximately 15 g of extra protein and the equivalent of approximately 216 extra kcal derived from carbohydrates and fat.

Body composition studies have shown that at term a rat fetus contains approximately 0.456 g of protein and 0.093 g of fat. For an average number of 10 fetuses per litter, the total amount of protein deposited in an entire litter would be 4.56 g. Adding to this figure the 0.106 g of protein deposited in each placenta (1), we find the total accumulation of protein in the product of conception to be approximately 5.62 g. Because of inefficiencies in digestion, a small percentage of the protein ingested by the mother is probably not absorbed. Even when this is considered, a comparison between the quantity of protein deposited in the conceptus (5.6 g) and the extra protein ingested by the mother (15 g) seems to demonstrate a maternal protein intake disproportionately larger than fetal needs. Although the cumulative energy requirements of the fetus are unknown, it is likely that a similar comparison will reveal that calories also are ingested far in excess of fetal energy needs.

Studies have demonstrated that species other than the rat, including the human, also ingest extra quantities of food during gestation. For example, studies of middle class women in England and the United States have shown that the average daily intake of calories and protein during pregnancy was more than 300 kcal and 35 g, respectively, above average daily prepregnancy levels (3). These increments represent a minimum cumulative extra intake of approximately 84,000 kcal and 9800 g of protein (included in the calorie count) over nonpregnancy levels. As in the rat, even after accounting for all the possible maternal losses, these extra quantities of ingested protein seem to be far in excess of the 543 g of protein accumulated at term in the fetus and the placenta, and the estimated 382 g of protein deposited in the uterus and the mammary gland or present in the expanded pool of circulating protein (3).

There is evidence that in addition to ingesting an excess of nutrients, pregnant animals also utilize certain nutrients, such as amino acids, more efficiently. For example, pregnant rats have a reduced rate of urea synthesis and reduced hepatic levels of certain catabolic enzymes, such as argininosuccinate synthetase and alanine-amino transferase (4, 5). The overall result of these changes is an increased protein utilization (6).

In the rat the deposition of protein and fat in the maternal carcass is only during the second week or second trimester of gestation, respectively (2, 3). At this time the maternal increments in food intake are clearly disproportionate to fetal needs since the fetus is only a small fraction of the total maternal weight. The maternal body handles this disproportion by depositing the excess of nutrients, largely protein and fat, in the maternal tissues. This accumulation of fat and protein is generally referred to as "maternal stores."

In the rat the deposition of protein and fat in the maternal carcass is noticeable as early as day 8 of gestation (4). It is not clear, however, whether the deposit occurs in a certain sequence and what proportion of such stores is used during the course of pregnancy. According to one source, the composition of the carcass at term is similar to that of a non-pregnant animal, which suggests that all the extra stores are utilized by the mother and the fetus (4). There are data, however, indicating net increments of 35 to 45% of fat and 0.5 to 1.5% of protein in the maternal carcass over the nonpregnancy levels (1).

The organ distribution of the protein deposited during pregnancy in the rat has been described as varying (7). For example, until day 14 of pregnancy most of the extra protein is present in muscle. At day 21 of gestation, however, most of the accumulated protein is present in liver. Such a shift reflects a net decrease in the amount of extra protein deposited in muscle and a net increase in liver (Table 1). According to these data, at term there would be a net gain in the maternal body of aproximately 220 mg of nitrogen or 1.37 g of protein. Thus, after delivery rats would have an excess store of both protein and lipids. The changes in the size and distribution of "maternal stores" of protein and lipids during gestation in the rat have been interpreted as reflecting "anabolic" and "catabolic" phases of pregnancy (1, 2). Such phases would coincide with two different periods of fetal growth. The anabolic phase, when protein stores are deposited, would comprise the first two weeks of gestation. As previously mentioned, during this period of pregnancy

Table 1 Distribution in Maternal Tissues of Nitrogen Retained by the Mother during Pregnancy[a]

	At Day 14	%	At Day 21	%
Total gain	616.3	100	220.3	100
Carcass (muscle)	500.5	81.2	60.0	27.2
Liver	85.6	13.8	125.1	56.7
Other tissues[b]	30.8	4.9	35.2	15.9

[a] Calculated from data by Naismith (7).
[b] Intestine, kidneys, spleen.

the fetus is still relatively small and its demands are minimal. The catabolic phase would take place during the last third of pregnancy, when fetal demands are presumably the highest. During the catabolic phase the mother would mobilize her extra stores of mainly muscle protein to ensure that fetal needs are met.

During the first two "anabolic" weeks, fat storage would be increased. Such a phenomenon would be reflected by an increased conversion of glucose into fatty acids and a diminished release of free fatty acids from the adipose tissue (2). By contrast, during the last week of gestation, the catabolic phase, adipose tissue fatty acid formation would decline to one-third of nonpregnancy levels and maternal fat stores would be increasingly mobilized as free fatty acids (2, 8, 9).

The changes in adipose tissue metabolism would be caused mainly by maternal hyperphagia and the peripheral response of adipose tissue to insulin (2). Thus, hyperinsulinism and excess food intake would promote the fat storage that takes place during the first two weeks. Later, because of diminished tissue responsiveness to insulin, maternal fat storage would decline. The anabolic phase of protein metabolism would be caused by increased levels of progesterone and the effect would be mediated through a reduced secretion of corticosteroids (1). In support of such a possibility it has been shown that progesterone administration in the rat causes a signficant reduction in the weight of the adrenal gland and lowers the plasma concentration of corticosteroids (9).

The catabolic phase of pregnancy would be regulated by levels of estrogen. Increased secretion of estrogen by the feto-placental unit during the last part of pregnancy would stimulate the synthesis of corticosteroids by the maternal adrenal gland by influencing ACTH secretion. The corticosteroids would, in turn, initiate and maintain maternal muscle protein catabolism (7). There is evidence that supports this possibility. The increase of plasma levels of estriol and corticosteroids during gestation parallels increments in the weight of the conceptus (10, 11). In the rat, administration of estradiol benzoate enhances synthesis and secretion of ACTH (12), while injections of cortisone cause a loss of protein from the carcass and a gain in liver protein (13). The same changes in the distribution of body protein have been seen to occur during the last week of pregnancy.

Current knowledge of the changes in maternal body composition during pregnancy in humans is still fragmentary. Based on analysis of tissue composition it has been determined that a total of 925 g of protein is deposited in the conceptus. This quantity represents an average daily gain of 3.3 g of protein. Because of the changing rates of fetal growth, however, protein will not be deposited in the fetus at a steady rate but rather at increasing quantities of 0.6, 1.8, 4.8, and 6.1 g/day during successive quarters of gestation (3). However, balance studies have demonstrated an average daily retention of nitrogen during pregnancy that is approximately three times higher than the theoretical average. After correcting for nitrogen losses in sweat, hair, nails, and so forth, daily body retention would be 1.1 g/day or 6.25 g of protein, which is still twice the theoretical calculations (14). Therefore, these studies would indicate that a significant deposit of protein occurs in maternal tissues.

This possibility, however, has been questioned (3). The main objection to the theory of a significant protein accumulation in the maternal body during pregnancy is that such a deposit would necessarily be accompanied by a proportional retention of water. It has been found in dog liver that under varying nutritional conditions the average ratio of water to protein content is 4:3. If a similar ratio exists in humans, and it is maintained in other tissues besides liver, a gain of 1600 g of protein, which is approximately the protein retention suggested by the metabolic studies, would produce a retention of 6900 g of water (3). No evidence of fluid retention of such magnitude has been found in pregnant women. Thus, by exclusion, it has been concluded that in humans the 3300 g of dry weight that constitutes the maternal stores is composed entirely of lipids (3). Such theoretical considerations contrast with experimental data. For example, total body potassium determinations in young pregnant women have shown an accumulation of potassium greater than the estimated gains in the fetus and accessory tissues of pregnancy (15). Unfortunately, although the girls included in the study conceived four or more years after menarche, it is still possible that they may have experienced some increments in lean body mass due to growth. In fact, this possibility has been demonstrated in a more recent study done in older women, between 24 and 34 years old, in which the same authors have been able to demonstrate a retention of K^+ of a lesser magnitude than the one found in the younger group. Similarly, the degree of nitrogen retention was also smaller (16). Still, the values obtained in the adult group of women support the original claim that maternal lean body mass increases during pregnancy. A summary of findings from metabolic studies done in pregnant women is presented in Table 2.

Table 2 Rate of Nitrogen Retention during Pregnancy and Distribution of the Retained Nitrogen between Fetal and Maternal Tissues

	Theoretical[a]	Women < 20 Years[b]		Women > 20 Years[c]	
		Observed	Corrected for N_2 losses[d]	Observed	Corrected for N_2 losses[d]
Rate of retention, g per day					
10 weeks	0.10	1.70	1.20	—	
20 weeks	0.29	1.20	0.70	1.06	0.56
30 weeks	0.77	1.75	1.25	1.28	0.78
40 weeks	0.98	1.85	1.35	2.15	1.65
Average daily retention	0.53	1.57	1.07	1.49	0.99
Total nitrogen retention, g	148.00[a]		299.6[d]		277.2[d]
N_2 deposited in the conceptus, g	86[a]		86[a]		86[a]
N_2 deposited in the mother, g					
Uterus, mammary gland, blood	62[a]		62[a]		62[a]
Other tissues	0		151.6		129.2

[a] Adapted from Hytten and Leitch (3).
[b] Adapted from Calloway (14).
[c] Adapted from King (15).
[d] Unmeasured nitrogen losses estimated to be 0.5 g/day.

If the metabolic studies discussed above prove to be correct, only 50% of the maternal stores would be composed of lipids, with an average accumulation of approximately 1.6 kg of fat. Paradoxically, although the accumulation of body fat during pregnancy is undisputed, the evidence of the phenomenon is mainly indirect. In fact, body fat content has been estimated during pregnancy using body density and total body water data, although problems with the type of subjects used and the design of the studies make it very hard to draw any conclusion in terms of the magnitude of the depot (17, 18). There are even two studies that would indicate a loss of body fat during pregnancy, although these results have been questioned on the basis of methodological problems (19, 20).

The amount of fat deposited subcutaneously can be assessed from measurements of skinfold thickness. With this method it was observed in 84 normal pregnant women that subcutaneous adipose tissue thickness increases during pregnancy with a marked disparity in the rate of deposit of new fat in various areas (21). For example, deposits in regions such as the abdomen, the back, and the upper thighs increased 20 to 40% whereas others did not change. Interestingly, most of the increments occurred during the first 30 weeks of pregnancy, with little subsequent change.

Unfortunately, there is no way to derive any estimate of total fat deposited subcutaneously from skinfold measurements. If it were possible and if changes in total body fat during pregnancy could be accurately determined it would then be possible to determine where the fat is being deposited.

For example, in the rat a considerable degree of fat accumlation, approximately 35 to 40% over prepregnancy levels, takes place in the carcass and also to some degree in the liver (1). Furthermore, it has been shown in the rat that the amount of DNA of the dorsal fat pad does not change during pregnancy, suggesting that fat accumulates by increments in cell size and not cell number (22). Since different fat deposits are known to have somewhat different metabolic characteristics, the lipid deposited in different regions could have different implications for maternal-fetal exchange.

FETAL GROWTH AND PLACENTAL FUNCTION

In most eutherian species fetal growth, as measured by changes in fetal body weight, increases constantly throughout pregnancy with more rapid increments during the last half. Biochemical analysis of different organs from human fetuses has demonstrated that fetal growth is almost exclusively proliferative up to the 25th week of gestation and both hyperplastic and hypertrophic thereafter (23). Tissues engaged in rapid cell division have very high oxygen and substrate requirements. It is therefore conceivable that fetal oxygen and substrate requirements per unit of tissue mass are higher than in most maternal tissues. It is also conceivable that parallel to the reduction in the rate of cell division the amount of substrates required by the fetus and its energy consumption per unit of body mass decrease with advanced gestation. Since the fetus is getting larger, however, its overall requirements are likely to be greater near term. In the rat if fetal requirements parallel the weight curve, there would be an approximately fortyfold increase in requirements during the last third of pregnancy (24). In man, during an analogous period of time, fetal requirements would increase only fivefold (25).

Most of the changes that take place in the maternal organism to maintain a normal rate of fetal growth are directly or indirectly caused by placental hormones. This has been elegantly demonstrated in the rat by experiments in which removal of the fetuses, without injury to the placenta, did not significantly alter some of the expected changes in maternal body weight (26). The placenta is also directly responsible for maintaining fetal growth by transferring from the maternal circulation all the nutrients required by the fetus. Thus, placental function is probably the single most important variable in fetal-maternal exchange. Like the fetus, the human placenta initially grows by cell multiplication and later by increase in cell size. These phases of growth are reflected in linear increments in DNA, a measure of cell number, followed by increments in the protein/DNA ratio, a parameter of cell size. In contrast to other organs, however, due to the presence of a large syncytium, placental DNA content does not reflect real cells, but rather the number of nuclei, and the protein/DNA ratio reflects the amount of protoplasm per nucleus.

In rat placenta DNA content increases linearly until day 17 of gestation while protein content continues to increase at the same rate until term (27). These changes indicate that cell division ceases at day 17 and that from that date until term there is a progressive increment in the protoplasmic mass per cell.

In human placenta DNA synthesis seems to cease around the 35th or 36th week of gestation and, as in the rat, during the last period of gestation the placenta maintains a purely hypertrophic growth (28).

Thus the placenta, although essentially a fetal organ, grows proportionately earlier than the fetus. Because of this earlier growth, in several species the placenta is bigger than the fetus during a considerable portion of pregnancy and therefore its requirements are probably greater than those of the fetus. For example, in the sheep up to the 100th day of gestation (average length of gestation in the sheep is 140 days) the oxygen consumption of the placenta has been found to be higher than the total fetal oxygen consumption (29). Such a finding suggests the possibility that if early in pregnancy there is a reduced oxygen supply or nutrient supply the placenta may compete with the fetus. Theoretically, since they are two biologic systems attached sequentially in such a manner that all the elements going into the fetus must first cross the cytoplasm of the placenta, the possibility seems a reasonable one. However, no clear evidence for a phenomenon of this type has been provided.

Later on in pregnancy the rate of fetal growth considerably exceeds that of placental growth. In both the human and the rat this is reflected by a rapid increase in the fetal weight/placental weight ratio. Because of this changing relationship between the placenta and the fetus the placenta must increase many times the amount of substances transferred per gram of tissue into the fetus in order to meet fetal needs. This increase has recently been demonstrated in the rat during the last week of gestation (30).

In these studies ^{14}C-labeled AIB and D-glucose-1-H^3 were injected into the maternal circulation and the concentration of label was measured in placenta and fetuses removed 10 minutes later. It was found that the concentration of AIB in placental tissues increased considerably between days 14 and 21, indicating a higher capacity of the placenta to take up and concentrate this substance (Fig. 1). The concentration of AIB in fetal tissues also increased

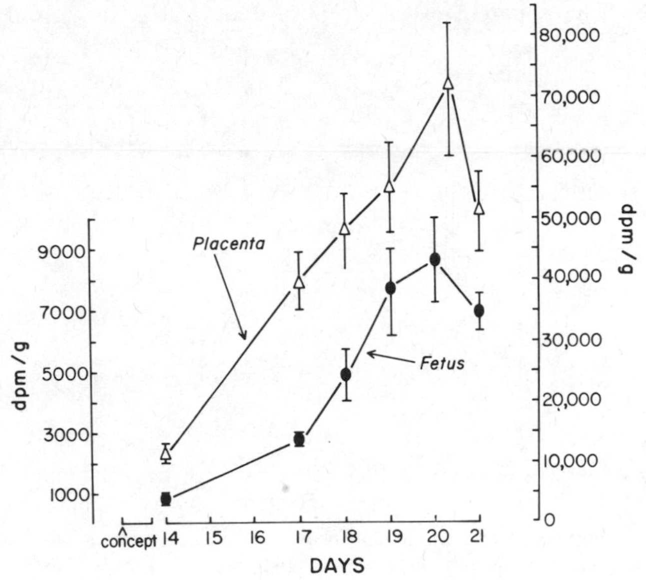

Figure 1. Concentration of AIB in placentas and fetuses removed 10 minutes after injection of AIB into the material circulation at different gestational ages (30).

proportionally to the placental changes, indicating that the quantity of AIB transported into the fetus is proportionally higher near term than in previous days. Whether similar changes occur with other amino acids is still unknown. During the last week of gestation the quantity of glucose transported into the fetus also increases proportionally more than increments in fetal weight (Fig. 2). Since glucose is probably transported across the placenta by facilitated diffusion, and AIB by active transport, the fact that during gestation the concentrations of both substances increase in the fetus suggests an overall increase in the ability of the placenta to transport these substances. It has been known, since pioneer work done almost three decades ago with labeled sodium, that rat placenta and placentas of other animals as well increase their "permeability" with advanced gestation (31). It was not known, however, that a similar phenomenon could take place for substances used in the oxidative metabolism of the fetus.

The seemingly disproportionate increments in placental transport described for glucose and AIB have not been observed for other nutrients such as ascorbic acid. In the rat, ascorbic acid is transported in quantities that are proportional to increments in fetal weight (32). Thus, concentration of labeled ascorbic acid per gram of fetal tissue, 10 minutes after injection of this vitamin into the mother, remains constant between 15 and 21 days of gestation (Fig. 3). The apparent excess of glucose and AIB transported into the

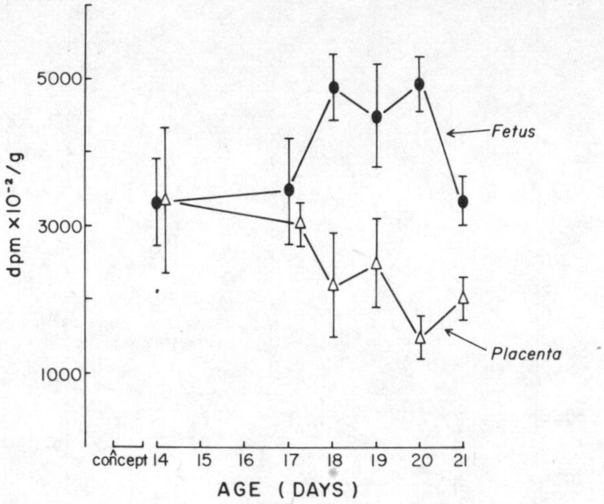

Figure 2. Concentration of label in placentas and fetuses removed 10 minutes after injection of D-glucose-1-H^3 into the maternal circulation at different gestational ages (30).

fetus can be interpreted as a safety measure to ensure that the fetus is receiving sufficient quantities of its two major nutrients.

In recent years evidence has been provided that at least in the human and in the fetal lamb, glucose and amino acids constitute the major source of calories. For example, in the sheep it has been estimated that glucose can supply at most only 50% of the substrate requirements of aerobic metabolism near term (33, 34). Furthermore, the contribution of amino acids to oxidative metabolism seems to be considerably higher than previous assumptions (35, 36).

MATERNAL-FETAL EXCHANGE DURING MATERNAL MALNUTRITION

A shortage of nutrients during pregnancy represents a serious and potentially dangerous situation for both the mother and the conceptus. If this situation

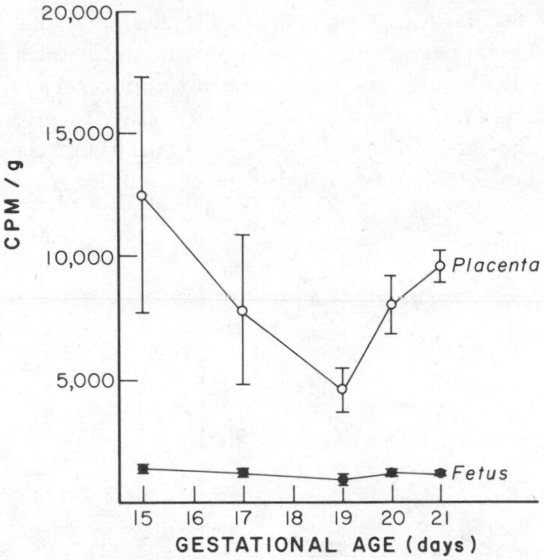

Figure 3. Concentration of label in placentas and fetuses removed 10 minutes after injection of absorbic acid-1-^{14}C) into the maternal circulation at different gestational ages (32).

is maintained long enough and at a significant degree of intensity, it may seriously disrupt the homeostatic mechanisms regulating normal maternal exchange. In all mammals in which the phenomenon has been studied, the effects of either an overall dietary restriction or a specific protein deficiency range from infertility to fetal death or various degrees of fetal growth retardation (37, 38).

In the rat most studies dealing with the effects of maternal malnutrition have utilized a 6% casein diet. The usual concentration of protein in laboratory rat diets ranges from 18 to 27%. In a typical experiment the animals are fed the low-casein diet at day 5 or 6 of pregnancy and are maintained on the diet until term. When compared with pregnant rats fed an adequate protein diet, the low-casein group gains considerably less body weight. In both groups, however, up to day 14 of pregnancy most of the weight gain represents increments in maternal components. As pregnancy advances, however, the weight of the conceptus becomes the major component; this situation is especially marked in the animals fed a 6% casein diet where the maternal component is measurable only until day 20 of gestation (39). Hence the increments in maternal body weight of the protein-malnourished rats between day 20 and term reflect solely the increments in the weight of the conceptus

(Fig. 4). The capacity of pregnant rats to accumulate maternal stores in spite of a nutrient deficiency is clear evidence of the greater efficiency in nutrient utilization that occurs during pregnancy. Furthermore, the subsequent decrease and final disappearance near term of maternal stores in the protein-malnourished animals supports the general assumption that the role of such stores is to help maintain fetal growth when nutrients are in short supply. In rats fed a low-casein diet fetal growth retardation becomes evident at day 14 of pregnancy (39). Since at this time the mother still has a significant

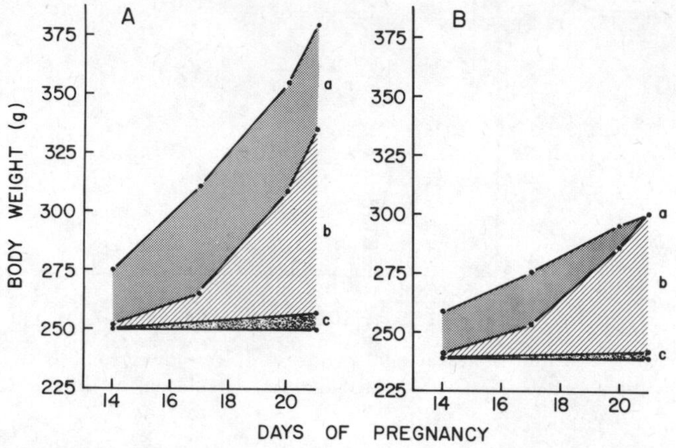

Figure 4. Components of body weight gain during pregnancy in animals fed a 27% (A) or 6% casein diet (B). In both groups (a) represents maternal body weight, (b) is the weight of the conceptus, and (c) are increments in body weight observed in non-pregnant animals of similar age and size fed a similar diet for the same length of time (39).

amount of extra weight the observation suggests that a shortage of protein affects fetal growth even before maternal stores are depleted. This would indicate that although the fetus has access to the maternal stores it is apparently unable to mobilize them. Such a possibility raises some questions about how nutrients are distributed between the maternal and fetal compartments. The current idea, based on Hammond's hypothesis, is that nutrients are normally distributed among tissues according to metabolic needs (40). Since the fetus is considered to have a higher metabolic rate than the maternal tissues, it would receive more nutrients per unit of body mass than the mother. Based on this hypothesis it was generally believed that the fetus was affected by maternal undernutrition only after all maternal stores, including prepregnancy stores, were depleted.

Hammond's hypothesis has been directly tested only once. In this test a group of pregnant rats were either underfed by an overall reduction in food intake or "overfed" by growth hormone administration along with a standard diet fed ad libitum (41). The results showed that changes in maternal body weight were proportional to the weight of the conceptus and to the levels of nutrient intake. These findings were interpreted to indicate that a certain minimum amount of nutrients is always supplied to the fetus and that any intake above this is distributed so that three-quarters goes to the conceptus and the remaining quarter goes to the mother.

Data from this study show, however, that body weight of rats fed 7 g day of diet, the most restricted group, was similar to prepregnancy levels. By contrast the weight of the conceptus in the same animal was markedly lower than controls. These results would indicate that if the fetus is indeed able to compete with the mother for available nutrients such a competition is limited to the pool of nutrients ingested in excess and stored during pregnancy and does not extend to those present in maternal tissues at conception.

A review of the data available in the literature demonstrates that in all mammalian species in which maternal malnutrition has been induced during pregnancy the loss of maternal body weight is proportionally less than the reduction in fetal body weight (Table 3). In the rat, a 50% reduction in dietary intake throughout pregnancy produces a 10% loss of maternal body weight (42). When diets are 75% restricted maternal losses in body weight range between 26 and 36% compared with initial body weight, while birthweight is reduced more than 50% (42).

In the guinea pig either a caloric or a protein restriction during the last half of pregnancy produces a significant increase in fetal mortality and approximately a 25% reduction in birthweight with no significant changes in maternal body weight (43). In the pig prolonged inanition during pregnancy causes an approximate 20% loss in maternal body weight compared with prepregnancy levels. Total embryonic nitrogen content, however, in the starved animals was 40% lower than controls (44). There is evidence that in certain subhuman primates and humans the same phenomenon occurs. For example, rhesus monkeys fed throughout gestation a diet containing only 25% as much protein as a control diet lose 0.4 kg from body tissues. This amounts to approximately a 7% loss of body weight. The mean birthweight of the neonates, however, decreased approximately 15% (45). Such a level of restriction produces some maternal deaths and a very high incidence of fetal losses due to abortion, stillbirth, and perinatal mortality.

Data collected during the Dutch famine also show a disproportionate effect of human maternal undernutrition on the conceptus. In this study mean values in maternal body weight, measured after delivery, decreased approximately 1% compared with the standard weight of nonpregnant women. During the same period of time birthweight decreased approximately 9% (46). In primates the birthweight reduction associated with maternal mal-

Table 3 Effect of Malnutrition during Pregnancy on Maternal and Fetal Body Weight in Some Mammalian Species. Values Represent Averages

	Maternal Weight (g)			Newborn Weight			
Species	Pre-pregnancy	Postpartum	Postpartum after malnutrition	Normal	After malnutrition	Type of Restriction	Source
Rat	215	+28g (+13%)[b]	−22g (−10%)	3.88g[a]	−0.45g (−12%)	50% dietary restriction	(42)
	215	+28g (+13%)[a]	−68g (−31.6%)	3.88g[a]	−1.99g (−51%)	75% dietary restriction	(42)
	240	+40g (+16.6%)	−18g (7.5%)	5.50g	−1.0g (−19%)	6% casein diet	(39)
Guinea pig	—	900	−93g (−10%)	78.5g	−21g (−28%)	Low protein (30% of control)	(43)
	—	900	−105g (−11.6%)	78.5g	−17g (−22%)	60% dietary restriction	(43)
Pig	116,000	+12,000g (+10%)	−28,000g (−24%)	289.9mg[c]	−135.8mg (−46.8%)	Total starvation for 34 days since mating	(44)
Macaca	5800	+1400g (+24%)	−400g (−6.9)	450g	−66g (−14.6%)	Low protein diet	(45)
Human	57,300	+7500g (+13%)	−600g (−1%)	3338g	−327g (−9%)	Approx. 40% calorie-protein restriction during last two-thirds of pregnancy	(46)

[a] Day 20 of gestation. [b] 34 days of pregnancy. [c] Lyophilized weight, mg.

nutrition is proportionately larger than the reduction in both body length and head circumference, which indicates that only a slight degree of fetal growth retardation is occurring (45, 46). By contrast, in rats and guinea pigs the reduction in birthweight reflects a proportional reduction in size and weight of all the organs.

Only a limited amount of information is available on changes in maternal body composition during dietary restriction. In a study done in rats fed different levels of protein it was found that a diet containing approximately 11% of casein produces a 5% loss in protein contents of the carcass and a 20% increase in protein content of the liver at term (1). In these animals there was a 15% reduction in protein content of the fetuses. This greater loss of protein content in the fetus is consistent with the idea that the mother is proportionally spared by malnutrition. However, the difference in nitrogen content of malnourished and control fetuses was found to be statistically nonsignificant.

More recent studies on body composition of rats fed a 5% casein diet during pregnancy have shown that, compared with nonpregnant animals fed a similar diet, the percentage of protein in the carcass does not change significantly while the percentage of body fat is higher (47) (Table 4).

Table 4 Effects of a 5% Casein Diet on Body Composition of Pregnant and Nonpregnant Rats

Group	% Protein	% Fat	% Water
Low protein (5% casein)			
nonpregnant	23.6	3.5	70.9
pregnant	22.8	6.7	68.5
Control (25% casein)			
nonpregnant	23.0	8.2	73.5
pregnant	21.8	12.3	66.1

[a] Adopted from Morgan (47).

Since in animals fed a 5% casein diet birthweight is reduced approximately 25%, it seems unquestionable that the fetus is proportionally more affected than the mother. Moreover, these results support the idea that when nutrients are in short supply the fetus is able to obtain from the mother only the extra stores accumulated during pregnancy. Thus, even in extreme conditions, the fetus would not be able to deplete the mother of either the protein or the fat present before pregnancy.

MATERNAL COMPARTMENTALIZATION

Based on the information discussed above the general conclusion can be drawn that in several mammalian species the pregnant mother is able to compartmentalize available nutrients. Indirect evidence for the existence of the phenomenon of maternal compartmentalization is provided by the fact that the amount of maternal reserves that can be mobilized during fasting largely exceeds the body loss that occurs after malnutrition during pregnancy. For example, a nonpregnant rat may easily lose more than 20% of its body weight after a few days of starvation (48). Although a high proportion of that loss is likely to be just body fluids, in a rat whose prepregnancy weight was 250 g a loss of even 10% of body weight would be sufficient to provide the amount of calories and protein needed by the fetus to maintain a normal growth rate. A similar example could be cited in humans, the difference being that the ratio of maternal weight to conceptus weight is greater in the human and, therefore, the percentage of maternal stores mobilized to maintain normal fetal growth would be even smaller. Assuming that the fetus is indeed more active metabolically than the maternal tissues and that based on this higher metabolic rate it could compete with the mother, there are two basic mechanisms by which the mother may avoid being depleted by the fetus. One mechanism would be to reduce fetal requirements by reducing either the metabolic rate of the fetus or its rate of growth. Such a possibility seems biologically unlikely to occur. Another possibility would be to reduce transfer of nutrients to the fetus. There are two ways by which this could be accomplished. One way would be to reduce uterine blood perfusion; another would be to reduce the ability of the placenta to transport nutrients. The increase in the amount of blood perfusing the uterus is one of the most important changes that occur during pregnancy. The maternal blood is the only source of oxygen and, except for the possibility of some protein ingestion from amniotic fluid late in pregnancy (49), it is also the only source of nutrients for the fetus. In man and other mammals, the percentage of the cardiac output delivered to the uterus increases during gestation proportionally to the increased fetal needs (3). The mechanisms regulating uterine blood flow are still unknown. As with other organs it is conceivable that still unknown local factors may have a role. However there is growing evidence which indicates that certain hormones, such as estrogens, may play an important role in influencing uterine blood flow (50, 51, 52). The effects of maternal malnutrition on estrogen synthesis and release are still unknown. A normal estriol excretion has been reported in pregnant women that were probably suffering from some degree of malnutrition (53). In starved pigs injections of estrogen and progesterone significantly increased the nitrogen content of the conceptus (44). It is not known, however, whether the effects of these hormones are mediated by an increased mobilization of maternal stores or increased uterine blood perfusion.

The possibility that the capacity of the placenta to transport nutrients may be reduced by maternal malnutrition is based on clinical and experimental evidence. Rats fed a low-protein diet from day 6 of pregnancy have smaller placentas at term, with a 25% lower protein and DNA content than placentas from a control group (54). These results suggest that the placenta is no exception to the principle that undernutrition interferes with hyperplastic growth (55).

Furthermore, since in rat placenta cell division proceeds until day 17 of gestation (27), the data suggest that the shortage of nutrients reaches a critical level before that day. The RNA content of these placentas has been found to be increased at day 13 of gestation (56). However, another study has demonstrated that at term placentas from protein-malnourished rats have a significant reduction in RNA content (54). Placental DNA content has been found to be significantly reduced in a population of poor women (57). Other studies done in similar populations have also found lower average values for DNA content compared with placentas delivered by women that presumably are better nourished (56, 58). However, the difference between groups was not statistically significant. The apparent discrepancies between these studies may be explained by factors such as sample size and differences in the nutritional status of the groups being compared. Total protein content has also been reported to be slightly but not significantly decreased in placentas from a malnourished population (58).

These results suggest that a moderate degree of maternal undernutrition, probably a caloric deficit, produces only a minor interference with the proliferative and hypertrophic phases of placental growth. Some parameters of RNA metabolism, however, seem to be more affected by a deficit of nutrients than DNA and protein content. For example, the polysome/monosome ratio has been found to be 50% lower in placentas from malnourished women (58). Polysomes consist of a strand of messenger RNA with ribosomes attached and are the basic units for protein synthesis. Two types of polysomes exist in the cell, those attached to the secretory membrane of the endoplasmic reticulum, or "bound polysomes," and those not associated with such a structure, or "free polysomes." For both populations of women the "bound polysomes" averaged 21% of the total number of ribosomes. This finding suggests a similar capacity to synthesize export proteins, conceivably peptide hormones, in the low socioeconomic, presumably undernourished, group. Further, in spite of the higher percentage of polysomal disaggregation, suggesting a reduced organ capacity to synthesize protein, cell-free protein synthesis per milligram of ribosomal RNA was similar in the malnourished and well nourished women. Thus, when the total capacities of the placentas for protein synthesis, obtained by multiplying in vitro amino acid incorporation per milligram of RNA content, were compared they were found to be similar in both populations. This finding would suggest that in spite of the reduced polysome/monosome ratio, maternal malnutrition would not reduce significantly the overall metabolic efficiency of the organ.

Further evidence of abnormal RNA metabolism has been provided by studies demonstrating elevated alkaline ribonuclease activity (RNase) in placentas of malnourished women when compared with a well-nourished population (59). The cellular role of this enzyme is still poorly understood. High levels of RNase are usually associated with an increased rate of RNA turnover (60, 61). A low-protein diet or dietary restriction has been shown to cause elevation of RNase in liver and brain in the rat. A protein-calorie supplementation during pregnancy has been found to reduce placental levels of RNase activity (62), suggesting that, out of the many variables that may influence placental metabolism, nutrition may have a direct influence on RNase activity.

The most substantial evidence that transfer of nutrients into the fetus is reduced by maternal malnutrition near term has been obtained recently in experiments done on rats fed a 6% casein diet. In these experiments 1 μci per 100 g of body weight of ^{14}C labeled AIB was injected into the maternal circulation at days 20 and 21 of gestation. Samples of maternal blood and one placenta were removed from each animal 10, 20, 40, and 60 minutes later. It was found that in malnourished animals the radioactive labeled amino acid had a lower rate of disappearance from the maternal plasma, stayed longer in the placenta, and was transported in reduced amount, to the fetuses (63) (Fig. 5).

In order to determine whether the reduced maternal-fetal transfer of AIB into the conceptus found in the protein malnourished animals reflected a a general reduction in the transfer of nutrients or was specific to AIB, maternal transfer of glucose and of a methyl-D-glucopyranoside (AMG), a nonmetabolizable glucose analog, was studied in a similar group of animals. In these experiments only 21-day pregnant animals were used and because of the pattern of placental transfer of glucose and AMG, only samples removed 10 minutes after maternal injection were used. It was found that in rats fed a 6% casein diet both substances were slightly increased in maternal plasma and significantly decreased in placentas and fetuses. The lower concentration in fetal tissues reflects a marked reduction in the amount of glucose and AMG transported to the fetuses per gram of placental tissue per minute (64) (Fig. 6).

In contrast to results obtained in rats, placental transfer studies done in protein- or caloric-restricted guinea pigs have shown that the amount of AIB transported into the fetus per gram of fetal weight was similar in controls and

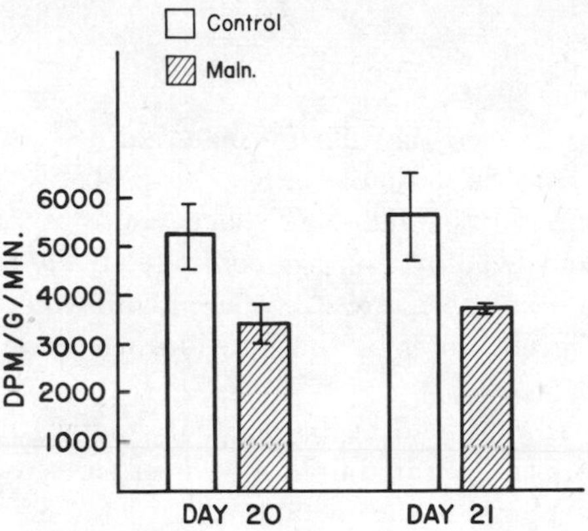

Figure 5. Quantity of AIB transferred into the fetuses per gram of placental tissue and per minute in control and protein-malnourished rats (63).

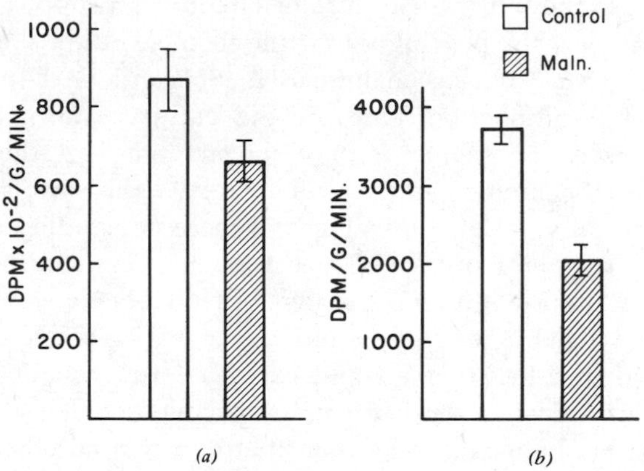

Figure 6. Amount of glucose (A) and AMG (B) transported into the fetus per gram of placental tissue per unit of time in malnourished and control rats (64).

calorie-restricted animals and increased in the protein-restricted ones (43). A possible interpretation of the apparent discrepancy between these two studies is that the guinea pig is more sensitive than the rat to nutrient deprivation. Thus, shortly after the onset of maternal malnutrition the nutrient supply to the fetus is drastically reduced. Supporting such an assumption is the fact that the restricted guinea pigs had a 50% fetal mortality. After such a marked reduction in fetal mass, transfer would continue at a reduced rate that may be proportional to fetal weight or, for unknown reasons, even higher per gram of fetal weight near term in the protein-restricted animals. In fact, if the elevated concentration of AIB in the protein-restricted pups represents a compensatory mechanism fetal weight should be less affected.

CONCLUSIONS

Evidence has been presented that during maternal malnutrition the mother is able to compartmentalize available nutritients probably by reducing blood perfusion to the uterus or by reducing placental transport of nutrients or both. Such mechanisms would begin to operate relatively early in pregnancy while pregnancy maternal stores are still present, and would prevent a serious depletion of the maternal stores by the fetus during the last stages of gestation.

The picture of maternal-fetal exchange that emerges from the data discussed here is far more complicated than the current idea that the main factor of maternal-fetal exchange is the metabolic rate of the maternal and fetal tissues. In fact, contrary to the idea of fetal parasitism, there seem to be feedback mechanisms operating in the mother that would reduce the maternal supply line to the fetus when nutrients are in short supply. From a teleological point of view the possibility that the mother, rather than the fetus, is proportionally spared during malnutrition seems to be a more plausible theory than the traditional one based on the fetal parasitism concept. In the mammalian species, pregnancy is only the first stage of the reproductive cycle. Lactation, beginning shortly after delivery, is in most species equally essential for the survival of the young and more demanding of the mother from a nutritional point of view. Thus it would seem a rather inadequate evolutionary adaptation if after a shortage of food a depleted mother were to deliver a normal baby that she is unable to care for. Nevertheless if a moderately malnourished mother must care for a runt, chances are that the mother will recover when food becomes available and will conceive again. This seems to be a better outcome than that of a normal offspring lactating from a malnourished mother, surviving, and eventually achieving sexual maturity.

REFERENCES

1. Naismith, D. J. The requirement for protein, and the utilization of protein and calcium during pregnancy. *Metabolism* **15**:582 (1966).
2. Knopp, R. H., Saudek, C. D., Avky, R. A., and O'Sullivan, J. B. Two phases of adipose tissue metabolism in pregnancy: maternal adaptations for fetal growth. *Endocrinology* **92:** 984 (1973).
3. Hytten, F. E. and Leitch, I. *The Physiology of Human Pregnancy*. Blackwell, Oxford, 1971.
4. Beaton, G. H., Beare, J., Ryu, M. H., and McHenry, E. W. Protein metabolism in the pregnant rat. *J. Nutr.* **54:** 291 (1954).

5. Naismith, D. J. Adaptations in the metabolism of protein during pregnancy and their nutritional implications. *Nutr. Rep. Intern* **7**:383 (1973).
6. Tagle, M. A., Ballester, D., and Donoso, G. Net protein utilization of a casein diet by the pregnant rat. *Nutr. Dieta.* **9**:21 (1967).
7. Naismith, D. J., The foetus as a parasite. *Proc. Nutr. Soc.* **28**:25 (1969).
8. Hamosh, M., Clary, T. R., Chernick, S. S., and Scrow, R. O. Lipoprotein lipase activity of adipose tissue and plasma triglyceride in pregnant and lactating rats. *Biochem. Biophys. Acta.* **210**:473 (1970).
9. Naismith, D. J. and Fears, R. B. Progesterone—the hormone of protein anabolism in early pregnancy. *Proc. Nutr. Soc.* **31**:79A (1972).
10. Ratanasopa, V., Schindler, A. E., Lee, T. Y., and Herrmann, W. L. Measurement of estriol in plasma by gas liquid chromatography. *Am. J. Obstet. Gynecol.* **99**: 295 (1967).
11. Baylis, R. I. S., Browne, J. C. M., Round, B. P., and Steinbeck, A. W. Plasma 17-hydroxycorticosteroids in pregnancy. *Lancet* **1**: 62 (1955).
12. Gemzell, C. A. Increase in the formation and secretion of ACTH in rats following the administration of oestradiol monobenzoate. *Acta Endocrinol.* **11**: 221 (1952).
13. Goodlad, G. A. J. and Munro, H. N. Diet and the action of cortisone on protein metabolism. *Biochem. J.* **73**: 343 (1959).
14. Calloway, D. H. Nitrogen balance during pregnancy In: *Nutrition and Fetal Development.* M. Winick, ed. Wiley, New York, 1974, pp. 79–94.
15. King, J. C., Calloway, D. H., and Margen, S. Nitrogen retention, total body ^{40}K and weight gain in teenage pregnant girls. *J. Nutr.* **103**:772 (1973).
16. King, J. C. Personal communication.
17. Seitchik, J., Alper, C., and Szutka, A. Changes in body composition during pregnancy. *Ann. N.Y. Acad. Sci.* **110**:821 (1963).
18. McCartney, C. P., Pottinger, R. E., and Harrod, J. P. Alterations in body composition during pregnancy. *Am. J. Obstet. Gynecol.* **77**:1038 (1959).
19. Flanagan, B., Muldowney, F. P., and Cannon, P. J. The relationship of circulating red cell mass, basal oxygen consumption and lean body mass during normal human pregnancy. *Clin. Sci.* **30**:439 (1966).
20. Seitchik, J. and Alper, C. The estimation of changes in body composition in normal pregnancy by measurement of body water. *Am. J. Obstet. Gynecol.* **71**:1165 (1956).
21. Taggart, N. R., Holliday, R. M., Billewicz, W. Z., Hytten, F. E., and Thompson, A. M. Changes in skinfold during pregnancy. *Brit. J. Nutr.* **21**:439 (1967).
22. Knopp, R. H., Herrera, E., and Freinkel, N. Carbohydrate metabolism in pregnancy. VIII. Metabolism of adipose tissue isolated from fed and fasted pregnant rats during late gestation. *J. Clin. Invest.* **49**:1438 (1970).
23. Widdowson, E. M., Crabb, D. E., and Milver, R. D. G. Cellular development of some human organs before birth. *Arch. Dis. Child.* **47**:652 (1972).
24. Rosso, P. Unpublished observations.
25. Lubchenko, L. O., Hausman, C., Dressler, M., and Boyd, E. Intrauterine growth as estimated from live-born birth weight data at 24–42 weeks of gestation. *Pediatrics* **32**: 793 (1963).

16. Bourdel, G., and Jacquort, R. Rôle du placenta dans les facultés anabolisantes des Rattes gestantes. *Concept. Rend. Acad. Sci.* **242**:552 (1956).

27. Winick, M. and Noble, A. Quantitative changes in DNA, RNA and protein during prenatal and postnatal growth in the rat. *Nature* **212**:34 (1966).

28. Winick, M., Coscia, A., and Noble, A. Cellular growth of human placenta. I. Normal placental growth. *Pediatrics* **39**:248 (1967).

29. Rosenfeld, C. R., Morris, F. H., Jr., Makowski, E. L., Meschia, G., and Battaglia, F. C. Circulatory changes in the reproductive tissues of ewes during pregnancy. *Gynecol. Invest.* **5**: 252 (1974).

30. Rosso, P. Changes in the transfer of nutrients across the placenta during normal gestation in the rat. *Am. J .Obstet,* **122**:2761 (1975).

31. Flexner, L. B. and Gellhorn, A. The comparative physiology of placental transfer. *Am. J. Obstet. Gynecol.* **43**: 965 (1942).

32. Rosso, P. and Norkus, E. Prenatal aspects of ascorbic acid metabolism in the albino rat. *J. Nutr.* **106**:767 (1976).

33. Boyd, R. D. H., Morris, F. H., Jr., Meschia, G., Makowski, E. L., and Battaglia, F. C. Growth of glucose and oxygen uptakes by fetuses of fed and starved ewes. *Am. J. Physiol.* **225**:897 (1973).

34. James, E., Raye, J. R., Gresham, E. L., Makowski, E. L., Meschia, G. and Battaglia, F. C. Fetal oxygen consumption, carbon dioxide production, and glucose uptake in a chronic sheep preparation. *Pediatrics* **50**:361 (1972).

35. Morris, F. H., Jr., Makowski, E. L., Meschia, G., and Battaglia, F. C. The glucose/oxygen quotient of the term human fetus. *Biol. Neonate* **25**:44 (1975).

36. Gresham, E. L., Simons, P. S., and Battaglia, F. C. Maternal-fetal urea concentration difference in man: metabolic significance. *J. Pediat.* **79**:809 (1971).

37. Giroud, A. Nutrition of the embryo. *Fed. Proc.* **27**:163 (1968).

38. Moustgaard, J. Nutritive influences upon reproduction. *J. Reprod. Med.* **8**:1 (1972).

39. Rosso, P. Maternal-fetal exchange during protein malnutrition in the rat. Changes in maternal and conceptus weight. *J. Nutr.* (in press).

40. Hammond, J. Physiological factors affecting birth weight. *Proc. Nutr. Soc.* **2**:8 (1944).

41. Frazer, J. F. D. and St. G. Huggett, A. The partition of nutrients between mother and conceptuses in the pregnant rat. *J. Physiol.* **207**:783 (1970).

42. Berg, B. N. Dietary restriction and reproduction in the rat. *J. Nutr.* **87**:344 (1965).

43. Young, M. and Widdowson, E. M. The influence of diets deficient in energy, or in protein, on conceptus weight, and the placental transfer of a non-metabolisable amino acid in the guinea pig. *Biol. Neonate* **27**:184 (1975).

44. Anderson, L. L. Embryonic and placental development during prolonged inanition in the pig. *Am. J. Physiol.* **229**:1687 (1975).

45. Kohrs, M. B., Harper, A. E., and Kerr, G. R. Effects of a low-protein diet during pregnancy of the rhesus monkey. I. Reproductive efficiency. *Am. J. Clin. Nutr.* **29**:136 (1976).

46. Stein, Z., Susser, M., Saenger, G., and Marolla, F. Famine and Human Development. The Dutch Hunger Winter of 1944/45, Oxford, New York, 1975.

47. Morgan, B. O. G. Effects of prenatal and postnatal undernutrition in the rat. Ph.D. thesis, University of London, 1975.

48. Arora, D. J. S. and deLamirande, G. The influence of starvation on rat liver polysomes. *Can. J. Biochem.* **49:**1150 (1971).

49. Pitkin, R. M. and Reynolds, W. A. Fetal ingestion and metabolism of amniotic fluid protein. *Am. J. Obstet. Gynecol.* **123:**356 (1975).

50. Greiss, F. C., and Anderson, S. G. Effect of ovarian hormones in the uterine vascular bed. *Am. J. Obstet. Gynecol.* **107:**829 (1970).

51. Greiss, F. C. and Martson, E. L. The uterine vascular bed: Effect of estrogens during ovine pregnancy. *Am. J. Obstet. Gynecol.* **93:**720 (1965).

52. Huckabee, W. E., Grenshaw, C., Ceiret, L. B., Mann, L., and Barron, D. H. The effect of exogenous estrogen on the blood flow and oxygen consumption of the uterus of the non-pregnant ewe. *Quart. J. Exp. Physiol. Cog. Med. Sci.* **55:**16 (1970).

53. Iyenpar, L. Urinary estrogen excretion in undernourished pregnant Indian women. *Am. J. Obstet. Gynecol.* **102:**834 (1968).

54. Rosso, P., Wasserman, M., Rozovski, S. J., and Velasco, E. Effects of maternal undernutrition on placental metabolism and function. In The Neonate. D. S. Young, and J. M. Hicks, Eds. Wiley, New York, 1976.

55. Winick, M., and Noble, A. Cellular response in rats during malnutrition at various ages. *J. Nutr.* **89:**300 (1966).

56. Winick, M. Cellular growth of the placenta as an indicator of abnormal fetal growth. In Diagnosis and Treatment of Fetal Disorders. K. Adamsons, Ed., Springer-Verlag, New York, 1969, pp. 83–101.

57. Dayton, D. H., Filer, L. J., and Canosa, C. Cellular changes in placentas of undernourished mothers in Guatemala. *Fed. Proc.* **28:**488 (1966). (Abstr.)

58. Lapa, E. M., Driscoll, S. G., and Munro, H. N. Comparison of placentas from two socioeconomic groups. II. Biochemical characteristics. *Pediatrics* **50:**33 (1972).

59. Velasco, E., Rosso, P., Brasel, J. A., and Winick, M. Activity of alkaline ribonuclease in placentas of malnourished women. *Am. J. Obstet. Gynecol.* **123:**637 (1975).

60. Girija, N. S., Pradham, D. S., and Sreenivasan, A. Effect of protein depletion on ribonucleic acid metabolism in rat liver. *Indian Biochem. J.* **2:**85 (1965).

61. Quinn-Stricker, C., and Mandel, P. Etude du renouvellemont du RNA des polysomes, du RNA de transfert et du RNA "messager" dans le foie de rat soumis a un jeune proteique. *Bull. Soc. Chim. Biol.* **50:**31 (1968).

62. Lechtig, A., Rosso, P., Delpado, H., Bassi, J., Martorell, R., Yarborough, C., Winick, M., and Klein, R. E. Effects of moderate maternal malnutrition on the levels of alkaline ribonuclease activity of the human placenta (submitted for publication) 1976.

63. Rosso, P. Maternal-fetal exchange during protein malnutrition in the rat. Transfer of α amino isobutyric acid. *J. Nutr.* (in press) 1976.

64. Rosso, P. Maternal-fetal exchange during protein malnutrition in the rat. Transfer of glucose and methyl (α-D-U-14 C glucose) pyranoside. *J. Nutr.* (in press) 1976.

2

Nutrition during Pregnancy: the Clinical Approach

ROY M. PITKIN, M.D.

Department of Obstetrics and Gynecology, University of Iowa, Iowa City, Iowa

The relationships between nutrition and pregnancy are exceedingly complex and poorly understood. The clinician, in attempting to integrate and apply basic scientific observations to patient care, faces several sources of frustration. Chief among these is that nutrition in the human rarely if ever constitutes an isolated variable. Rather it occurs as part of a cluster of circumstances of social, economic, cultural, and geographic natures. Even when nutrition can be identified as a specific variable, delineation of the precise roles played by individual nutrients is almost impossible. Thus, interpretation of epidemiologic data is seriously hindered by an inability to separate nutrition from other confounding influences and an inability to assess the relative contributions of individual nutrients.

Many of the data regarding nutritional influences on human pregnancy have been based on the observed correlation between maternal and infant weights. Numerous studies have indicated that maternal weight gain during pregnancy and, to a lesser extent, maternal prepregnant weight correlate independently with infant weight at birth. To be sure, maternal weight and weight gain are crude indices of nutrition, and birthweight is a similarly crude index of fetal development. Nevertheless, weight represents a simple and objective measurement and a positive correlation between maternal and newborn weights almost surely indicates the importance of nutritional influence on the course and outcome of pregnancy.

SPECIFIC NUTRIENTS

Energy, Weight, and Weight Gain

Additional energy sources needed during pregnancy are related to the added tissues and increased metabolism of the pregnant woman as well as to the growth of the conceptus. The total energy cost of pregnancy, calculated from the amounts of protein and fat accumulated by the mother and fetus and the additional metabolism incurred by these tissues, amounts to approximately 75,000 kcal (1). Caloric expenditure is relatively constant throughout the last two-thirds of gestation, with the extra caloric cost of the second trimester related principally to the maternal compartment and that of the third trimester mainly to the fetal compartment. Dividing the total additional energy cost of pregnancy by the duration of gestation yields a daily increment of 300 kcal per day, which represents an addition of approximately 15% to the Recommended Dietary Allowance (2) for energy in the mature "reference" woman. These levels relate to the needs for pregnancy and do not take into account such variables as physical activity, ambient temperature, or growth requirements unrelated to gestation.

The simplest method of assessing energy intake is observation of pregnancy weight gain. While *total* weight gain during gestation has been the focus of much attention, the *pattern* by which weight accumulates is of greater significance. The usual pattern consists of minimal gain (1 to 2 kg) during the first trimester and a progressive linear rate of gain averaging 350 to 400 g per week through the last two-thirds of gestation (3). Such a course will result in a mean total gain of 10 to 12 kg by term, but the pattern is more important than the total amount. These relationships, along with the components of the accumulation as a function of time, are illustrated in Fig. 1. During the second trimester most of the gain involves the maternal compartment (blood volume increase, uterine and breast growth, and fat storage) while that of the third trimester relates principally to the fetus, placenta, and amniotic fluid. Based on these considerations, it would be anticipated that the correlation between maternal nutrition and birthweight would be strongest when based on weight gain during late pregnancy. Such a relationship has been confirmed by studies demonstrating that the effects of maternal undernutrition on infant size are most marked when deprivation occurs during the third trimester (4, 5).

Prepregnant weight and pregnancy weight gain exert independent and additive influences on birthweight, relationships recently reviewed by Jacobson (6). Epidemiologic studies indicate that together they account for almost all of the observed variation at any given gestational age. Field studies

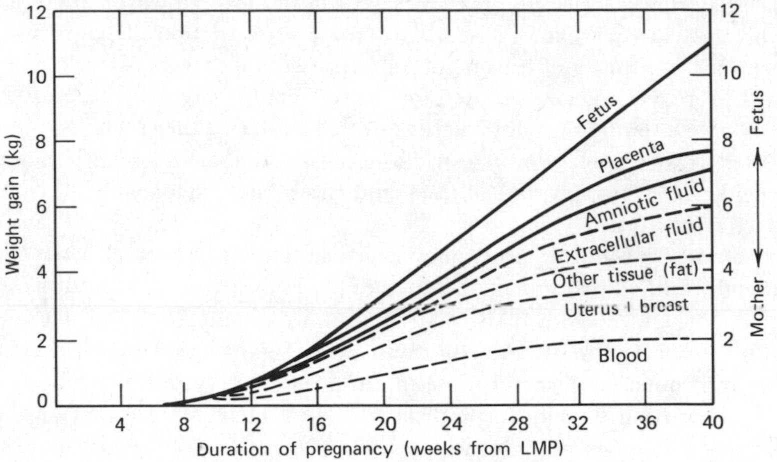

Figure 1. Average pattern and components of maternal weight gain during pregnancy. Reproduced with permission from *Nutritional Support of Medical Practice* (3).

involving provision of nutritional supplements to pregnant women of known or presumed deficient nutritional status indicate that such programs are associated with significant increases in birthweight. While nearly all investigations of the effect of nutrition on human pregnancy have focused on birthweight as the outcome variable, length, head circumference, and placental weight appear to be affected in the same manner as birthweight (5).

Deviations in weight and weight gain constitute common problems in clinical obstetric practice. The following definitions have been suggested as guidelines (3):

UNDERWEIGHT	prepregnant weight 10% or more below standard weight for height and age.
OVERWEIGHT	pre-pregnant weight 20% or more above standard weight for height and age.
INADEQUATE GAIN	gain of 1 kg or less per month during second or third trimesters.
EXCESSIVE GAIN	gain of 3 kg or more per month.

The *underweight* obstetric patient faces a number of hazards, principally that of a low birthweight infant. Studies have indicated improved outcome in these patients with a program involving protein-calorie supplements to correct past nutritional deficits as well as to provide for pregnancy (7). The *obese* pregnant patient is at increased risk for several complications, notably those associated with chronic hypertensive-vascular disease and diabetes mellitus (8). Restriction of gain has been widely advocated in these patients so that they might conclude pregnancy with a net loss. However, there is no convincing evidence that weight loss or marked restriction of gain in such patients has a salutary effect on the obstetric complications associated with obesity. Moreover, dietary restriction to limit energy often involves restriction of other essential nutrients such as protein. Finally, the catabolism of fat associated with severe caloric restriction results in ketone body production and evidence from several sources indicates that ketonemia is poorly tolerated by the fetus.

Inadequate gain during pregnancy is associated with increased risk of low birthweight with the attendant complications imposed by this condition. In addition, the patient with inadequate caloric intake may be subject to deficiencies of other nutrients. A subnormal rate of gain indicates the need for careful and intensive dietary counseling and follow-up assessment. *Excessive gain* has long been thought to predispose to a number of obstetric complications, especially preeclampsia, and several generations of American physicians have been raised on the concept that dietary restriction protects against the development of such conditions. Moreover, the definition of excessive weight gain has often been considerably more stringent (e.g., more than 16 or 18 pounds total gain) than that proposed here. Only in recent years has it been recognized that no cause-effect relationship exists between caloric intake (as reflected in weight gain) and preeclampsia. Energy intake above normal pregnancy needs will result in the deposition of excessive fat, which, if not lost at delivery, can contribute to the long-term development of obesity. Efforts to limit excessive gain may be advisable to prevent initiation of this chain of events but the aim of such efforts should be to bring the rate of gain near normal rather than to restrict it markedly.

Protein

Additional protein is needed during pregnancy for the expanded maternal plasma, uterus, and breasts, as well as for protein synthesis in the fetus and placenta. The magnitude of the pregnancy requirements, however, is uncertain since different methods used in estimation yield different values (9). Summation of the total amounts of known protein storage in the expanded maternal and fetal compartments and correction for efficiency of conversion from dietary to tissue protein yields a value of approximately 10 g per day in addition to the nonpregnant allowance. In contrast, experimental methods involving nitrogen balance studies usually result in estimates two or three times as great. The explanation of this apparent discrepancy is unclear at present but it has been suggested that it may reflect protein storage at unrecognized maternal sites such as muscle. The current philosophy seems to be to tentatively accept the higher allowance in view of uncertainties regarding protein storage during gestation. Accordingly, the Recommended Dietary Allowance for protein for the pregnant woman is 1.3 g/kg/day in the mature woman, 1.5 g/kg/day in the adolescent aged 15 to 18, and 1.7 g/kg/day in the girl under 15 (2).

The effects of protein deficiency in pregnancy are difficult to define precisely because of the inextricable metabolic relationships between energy and protein. A certain critical level of caloric intake is essential to "protect" protein from catabolism to meet basic energy requirements. Diets deficient in protein are usually also deficient in total energy content. Such difficulties notwithstanding, maternal protein intake seems to correlate positively with infant length and weight at birth (10). Some studies have also found an association between low protein intake (usually with low caloric intake as well) and preeclampsia (11).

The serum albumin concentration normally declines during pregnancy, reaching a nadir in the early third trimester, at which point the level is nearly 30% below the nonpregnant value. This adjustment appears to be physiologic in nature and under ordinary circumstances does not reflect protein intake (12). With marked protein deficiency, however, lower than normal levels may be encountered.

Iron and Folate

Pregnancy imposes a substantial burden on the maternal hematopoietic system (13). Plasma volume increases rapidly during early and middle pregnancy and then levels off in the last several weeks prior to term. At its maximum, the increase in plasma volume amounts to an average of 50% above the nonpregnant level. Erythrocyte volume increases in a more nearly linear manner, reaching a maximum (in patients not taking supplemental iron) of less than 20% above the nonpregnant level. To a considerable extent, iron represents the limiting factor in these hematologic adjustments since erythrocyte volume increases to nearly 30% above nonpregnant values when iron supplements are given. These relationships are illustrated in Fig. 2. The amount of elemental iron utilized in the augmented erythropoiesis of pregnancy with adequate iron available to the bone marrow is 500 mg. To this is added the iron content of the fetus and placenta (250 to 300 mg), making the "iron requirement" of pregnancy approximately 750 mg.

The potential sources available to meet the gestational iron needs include diet, stores, and supplementation. The usual American diet contains 10 to 15 mg of elemental iron daily, of which about 10% is absorbed. While absorption may increase at times of need (such as pregnancy), diet ordinarily provides no more than 2 or 3 mg/day, an amount similar to obligatory losses.

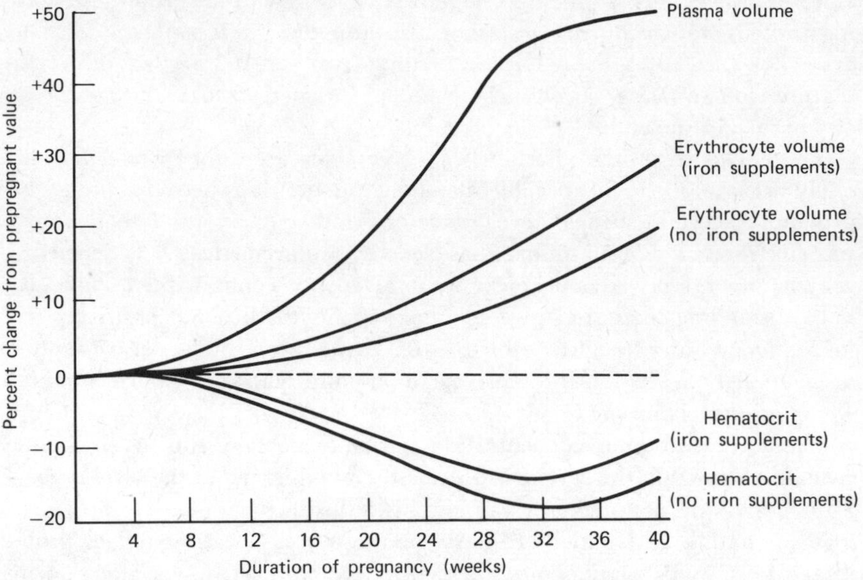

Figure 2. Changes in maternal plasma and erythrocyte volume during pregnancy. Reproduced with permission from *Nutritional Support of Medical Practice* (3).

Storage iron has been found to average 300 mg in healthy women and one-third of such subjects essentially lack iron stores in the reticulo-endothelial cells of the bone marrow. Thus, dietary and storage sources are generally inadequate to meet the iron needs of pregnancy and this nutrient is the one for which the need for routine supplementation seems most clearly established. The recommended level is 30 to 60 mg/day (14), an amount adequate to virtually eliminate iron deficiency anemia as a complication of pregnancy.

The principal effect of iron deficiency during pregnancy is maternal anemia. In unsupplemented patients, as many as one-half will have hemoglobin concentrations of 11 g/ml or less at term. In addition to the subjective symptoms associated with anemia, the patient with this complication is less able to tolerate hemorrhage and has greater propensity to infection. The fetal effects of maternal iron deficiency are surprisingly mild. Hemoglobin and iron levels in newborns typically bear no relation to maternal iron status, indicating the efficiency of the fetus in "parasitizing" this element from its mother (15).

Folate requirements are increased during pregnancy because of the augmented maternal erythropoiesis and the growth of fetal and placental tissues. The Recommended Dietary Allowance (2) for folate is 800 μg/day, which represents a doubling of the allowance for nonpregnant women. Megaloblastic anemia due to folate deficiency was first recognized in a pregnant woman and the majority of cases occur in association with gestation. Folate deficiency induces a sequence of biochemical and morphologic changes in the hematologic system and the incidence of deficiency depends on the diagnostic criteria used. Thus, low serum or erythrocyte folate levels are fairly common whereas anemia is relatively rare at least in contemporary American practice. Moreover, the clinical significance of preanemic indices of folate deficiency is unclear. While early retrospective studies suggested an association with spontaneous abortion, premature separation of the placenta, and pre-eclampsia, later and better designed studies have not been confirmatory (3).

The question of routine folate supplementation is controversial, in part because of the uncertain significance of preanemic indices of folate deficiency (13). The majority opinion appears to be that supplementation, while unnecessary as a routine, should be considered in instances in which the dietary assessment reveals a low intake or in those conditions (such as chronic hemolytic anemia, multiple pregnancy, or anticonvulsant drug therapy) in which needs are increased. If vitamins are to be supplemented at all, there is probably more reason to give folate than any other, particularly in view of dietary survey data indicating a marginal folate content of many American diets. Amounts of 400 to 800 μg/day appear appropriate for supplementation.

Infants born to women with megaloblastic anemia typically have normal hemoglobin levels, indicating that for folate, as for iron, the fetus is an effective parasite (16).

Calcium and Vitamin D

The calcium content of the fetal skeleton averages 30 g, with most of the accumulation occurring during the last trimester (17). In addition, some evidence suggests that calcium is stored in the maternal skeleton during pregnancy, perhaps in anticipation of lactation needs. The Recommended Dietary Allowance (2) for calcium in pregnancy is 1200 mg, an increase of 400 mg over the allowance for the nonpregnant woman. This intake should provide adequate amounts, particularly in view of the adaptive ability to increase absorption and decrease excretion at times of increased need. To be sure, a huge reservoir of calcium in the maternal skeleton is available and this probably explains why substantially lower calcium intakes accompany pregnancy in many cultures without catastrophic sequelae. Nevertheless, deficient calcium intake during pregnancy can apparently result in osteomalacia in the mother (18) and radiographic evidence of decreased bone density in the infant (19).

Vitamin D, either ingested in food or formed in the skin by the action of ultraviolet light on dehydrocholesterol, is essential in calcium metabolism. It facilitates intestinal absorption of calcium and, in concert with parathyroid hormone, promotes bone resorption. Vitamin D requirements do not appear to be increased markedly in pregnancy and the Recommended Dietary Allowance (2) is 400 IU/day for both pregnant and nonpregnant adults. In addition to its role in promoting a positive calcium balance during gestation, recent evidence suggests that the vitamin may play a role in neonatal calcium homeostasis. Vitamin D and its metabolites cross the placenta freely and low plasma levels have been found in some instances of early neonatal hypocalcemia (20), suggesting that maternal vitamin D deficiency in late pregnancy may be responsible for this complication. At the opposite extreme, a possible association of maternal hypervitaminosis D and the severe form of infantile hypercalcemia is suggested by epidemiologic observations and animal studies (21).

Other Vitamins and Minerals

Virtually all other vitamins and minerals are needed in modestly increased amounts during pregnancy. Generally, the levels required can be provided readily by diet. The traditional practice of prescribing vitamin-mineral supplements for the pregnant woman is thus probably unnecessary. Among the disadvantages of routine supplementation are cost and the potential for a false sense of security regarding nutritional status. On the other hand, the practice is not dangerous as long as toxic overdoses are avoided and it should therefore be viewed as an option.

CLINICAL APPROACH

Given the proposition that attention to nutrition represents an essential component of prenatal care, an official policy of the American College of Obstetricians and Gynecologists (22), the responsibility of the clinician is to ensure that each pregnant woman receives an assessment of nutritional status, dietary advice consistent with that assessment, and follow-up to evaluate the impact of the advice.

At the first prenatal visit a relatively formal assessment should be done, including history (specifically dietary history), complete physical examination, and laboratory studies. Included in these studies, as a minimum, should be a measurement of hemoglobin or hematocrit or both and a complete urinalysis. On the basis of this assessment at the initial prenatal visit, the degree of "nutritional risk" is estimated and advice given. The advice should be reasonably detailed and specific, yet expressed in terms understandable to the patient, and should take into account physiologic, cultural, and individual characteristics.

Certain findings in history, physical examination, and routine laboratory studies constitute nutritional risk factors and indicate a need for careful nutritional evaluation and advice. Examples of such conditions are

1. Obstetric history of preeclampsia, pregnancy loss, premature labor, low birthweight infant, or anemia.
2. Maternal alcoholism, smoking, drug addiction, or pica.
3. Extremes of age and parity.
4. Chronic maternal diseases such as hypertension, diabetes, cardiac or renal disease.
5. Abnormalities of weight prior to or during pregnancy.
6. Anemia, glucosuria, or ketonuria.

In addition to dietary counseling consistent with recognized standards, consideration should be given to nutritional supplementation. For practical purposes, all pregnant women should receive supplemental iron. It may be given in the form of simple ferrous salts, 30 to 60 mg/day throughout pregnancy and for two to three months postpartum. Supplemental folate may be given to all patients or, alternatively, to those in whom nutritional assessment indicates a low folate intake which cannot be corrected by dietary means, those with multiple pregnancy or chronic hemolytic anemia, and those taking anticonvulsants. Other vitamin-mineral supplements are considered optional.

Subsequent prenatal visits should include a brief follow-up dietary history and counseling as indicated. The pattern of weight should be assessed as an index of caloric intake, with gains of more than 3 kg per month or less than 1 kg in any month after the first trimester indicating a need for more careful attention. Urine testing should be repeated at intervals and hemoglobin-hematocrit should be measured early in the third trimester.

At the postpartum visit, the nutritional status should be reassessed and advice given for the interconceptional period. Implications with respect to nutrition in relation to lactation and various contraceptive techniques should be considered at this time.

REFERENCES

1. Hytten, F. E., and Leitch, I. *The Physiology of Human Pregnancy*. Blackwell, Oxford, 1971.

2. Food and Nutrition Board, *Recommended Dietary Allowance*, 8th edition. National Academy of Sciences, Washington, D.C., 1974.
3. Pitkin, R. M. In *Nutritional Support of Medical Practice*, C. E. Anderson, D. B. Coursin, and H. A. Schneider, Eds., Harper and Row, Hagerstown, 1975.
4. Naeye, R. L., Blane, W., and Paul, C. *Pediatrics* **52**:494 (1973).
5. Stein, Z., and Susser, M. *Pediatr. Res.* **9**:70 (1975).
6. Jacobson, H. N. *Clinics in Perinatology* **2**:233 (1975).
7. Higgins, A. C., Crampton, E. W., and Moxley, J. E. *Proceedings of the Fourth International Congress of Endocrinology*, 1972, p. 1071.
8. Peckham, C. H., and Christianson, R. E. *Am. J. Obstet. Gynecol.* **111**:1(1971).
9. King, J. C. *Clinics in Perinatology* **2**:243 (1975).
10. Burke, B. S., Harding, V. V., and Stuart, H. C. *J. Pediatr.* **23**:506 (1943).
11. McGanity, W. J., Cannon, R. O., Bridgforth, E. B., Martin, D. P., Densen, P. M., Newbill, J. A., McClellan, G. S., Christie, A., Peterson, J. C., and Darby, W. J. *Am. J. Obstet. Gynecol.* **67**:501 (1954).
12. Singh, H., Ramakumar, R., and Singh, I. D. *J. Obstet. Gynaecol. Brit. Cwlth.* **74**:254 (1967).
13. Kitay, D. Z., and Harbort, R. A. *Clinics in Perinatology* **2**:255 (1975).
14. Pitkin, R. M., Kaminetzky, H. A., Newton, M., and Pritchard, J. A. *Obstet. Gynecol.* **40**:773 (1972).
15. Rios, E., Lipschitz, D. A., Cook, J. D., and Smith, N. J. *Pediatrics* **55**:694 (1975).
16. Pritchard, J. A., Whalley, P. J., and Scott, D. E. *Am. J. Obstet. Gynecol.* **104**:388 (1969).
17. Pitkin, R. M. *Am. J. Obstet. Gynecol.* **121**:724 (1975).
18. Felton, D. J. C., and Stone, W. D. *Brit. Med. J.* **1**:1521 (1966).
19. Krishnamachari, K. A. V. R., and Iyengar, L. *Am. J. Clin. Nutr.* **28**:482 (1975).
20. Rosen, J. F., Roginsky, M., Nathenson, G., and Finberg, L. *Am. J. Dis. Child.* **127**:220 (1974).
21. Committee on Nutrition, American Academy of Pediatrics, *Pediatrics* **40**:1050 (1967).
22. American College of Obstetricians and Gynecologists: *Standards for Obstetric-Gynecologic Services*, 1974.

3

Nutrition and the Contraceptive Pill

DAPHNE A. ROE, M.D.

Division of Nutritional Sciences, Cornell University, Ithaca, New York

Hormonal methods of contraception have been used for almost 20 years, and it is estimated that approximately 50 million women are currently using these drugs in the world, and that 10 million of these are in the United States (1, 2). Four types of preparations have been used, but because of greater commercial availability and distribution, we have gained greatest experience of the effects of so-called combined preparations, in which each tablet of a 20- or 21-day course contains both an estrogen and a progestogen. Sequential products provide a course of tablets containing an estrogen only, followed by a short course of tablets containing both an estrogen and a progestogen. Other products that have been and are used include the "mini-pills", containing a low dose of a progestogen which is taken continually, and the depot contraceptives, in which either a progestogen alone or a mixture of progestogen and estrogen is given parenterally at intervals (3).

Within the different groups of oral contraceptives there is variability in the type and level of estrogen used as well as in the type and level of progestational agent. Two estrogens have been used, ethynyl estradiol, and the 3-methyl derivative of ethynyl estradiol, mestranol. Common progestogens used in the oral contraceptives (OC) have been derivatives of 19-nortestosterone, but in more recent years hydroxyprogesterone derivatives have also been employed. Knowledge of the differing composition and hormonal effects of oral contraceptives is necessary to our understanding of the metabolic consequences of taking these drugs and of their nutritional effects (4).

The primary mode of action of these drugs is to suppress ovulation. Estrogen-progestogen preparations suppress ovulation by influencing the release of gonadotropins from the pituitary gland. Inhibition of the release of follicle-stimulating hormone (FSH) and luteinizing hormone (LH) is due to the estrogen component but is apparently enhanced by the progestogen. Progestogens also affect the uterine endometrium, promoting shedding of this mucosa (1).

As is the case with endogenous sex steroids, contraceptive hormones affect carbohydrate, lipid, protein, mineral, and vitamin disposition. These drugs contain steroids, which are structurally similar to naturally occurring hormones, but they do not replicate the effects of the steroids normally present in the body, nor can it be said that the metabolic and nutritional effects of these drugs represent a condition of pseudopregnancy with the accompanying changes in hormonal status.

Since these drugs became widely available, many reports have suggested that they may have an adverse effect on nutritional status. Before we attempt to analyze these publications, we must remember certain basic facts. For example, because vitamin depletion may be induced in certain women by prolonged use of OC, it should not be inferred that all women receiving these drugs are similarly at risk. Even if we can show that OC or specific components of these drugs can cause adverse changes in nutritional status, there is much evidence to suggest that only certain women are vulnerable. The effects of these drugs on nutrient transport and utilization differ in such a way that only a few nutrients, mainly water-soluble vitamins, are actually depleted, and even among these nutrients the rate and level of depletion may be low. Only some women, then, are nutritionally at risk, and it is my purpose to identify who may be at risk and how nutritional status may be affected.

We should first note two important points: that the body may become adapted to the metabolic effects of these drugs, and that we are unable to predict the nutritional consequences of OC usage unless we are acquainted with the dietary intake of the user. Investigators have been particularly remiss in obtaining this information. We should not be satisfied that the nutritional effects of these drugs are trivial until we have investigated previously malnourished women and until we have thoroughly examined the information on the precise nutritional status of women who discontinue these drugs for medical reasons.

It has been emphasized by Doll and Vessey (5) that since oral contraceptives are so widely used, every type of disease that occurs normally among women of reproductive age would also be likely to occur among women who were taking these drugs. These authors suggest that it is therefore not surprising that many illnesses presumed to be adverse reactions to OC have been reported. In addition, some women receiving these drugs may not only be receiving marginal diets, but may also suffer preexisting conditions that increase or decrease their nutritional requirements.

CHANGES IN WEIGHT AND BODY CONTOUR

Nutritional problems attributed to contraceptive steroids tend to reflect or exaggerate slightly the nutritional problems of the community or population in which they occur. For example, in middle-aged women or younger women tending to obesity, weight gain is often blamed on OC and is considered a prominent side effect. The weight gain that properly can be associated with the intake of certain combination-type drugs is due either to fluid retention or to nitrogen retention, and was more usual when the drugs contained a high ostrogen component. Although an increase in abdominal girth has been described, Bakker and Dightman (6), in a study over a four-year period in which women were weighed at every visit, did not find a significant trend for weight gain or weight loss in their subjects. It was noted, however, that in a small group of women, when the drugs were discontinued, some 30% showed a decrease in weight of short duration, which might be suggestive of fluid loss.

In a health and nutrition survey that I conducted among 469 low-income rural women, 206 women had taken contraceptive steroids at one time or another, but only eight had actually discontinued these drugs because of weight gain, though others complained of this or some complication of OC use (7). In this group 61.5% of the women were defined as obese.

EVIDENCE OF ALTERED NUTRIENT REQUIREMENTS

Among the nutritional abberations that have been attributed to contraceptive steroid preparations, a reduction in serum and erythrocyte folacin levels has been amply documented. There have also been a few reports of megaloblastic anemia associated with folate deficiency. The first report of lowered serum folate levels in women taking these drugs was published in 1968 by Shojania and associates (8). These same investigators subsequently showed that erythrocyte folate levels might be substantially reduced in subjects taking OC and that additional biochemical evidence of folate deficiency or depletion might be obtained among these women (9). This group has subsequently contributed largely to our knowledge of women at risk for the development of folate depletion while taking these drugs. They have identified that whereas the majority of women taking OC absorb both the monoglutamic and polyglutamic forms of folate normally, there is a distinctive subgroup who show mild folate malabsorption. These investigators consider that evidence of malabsorption of folate with clear-cut evidence of deficiency may arise in women who have malabsorption syndromes which may not have previously been brought to light (10). More recently they found that women taking OC excreted more folate in their urine for any given level of serum or red cell folate, and they believe that the increased urinary folate excretion may in part explain lower serum and red cell folate levels in women taking these drugs (11). Their findings are in contrast to those of Streiff (12), who obtained some evidence that women taking these drugs are unable to absorb polyglutamic forms of folate as efficiently as control subjects. Streiff's findings on polyglutamate malabsorption are also contradicted by Stephens et al. (13), who found that provided subjects are presaturated with folic acid, there is no statistical difference in polyglutamate absorption between women taking OC and control subjects.

Certain important questions must be asked. Are there certain women, or groups of women, who are particularly at risk for the development of folate deficiency during prolonged intake of OC? How can these women be recognized? And how can we prevent the development of this nutritional impairment? Both survey data and case studies have indicated that the women at risk for folate depletion with use of these drugs include those on marginal intakes of the vitamin, women who consume alcohol excessively, those with malabsorption syndromes, those with other diseases conferring an increased folate requirement, and perhaps pregnant women who conceive shortly after discontinuing use of OC drugs (14).

While the literature is somewhat confusing about the relative level of red cell depletion induced by these drugs, it would appear that when homogeneous and comparable OC users and control subjects have been chosen for study, regardless of the folate status of the control group, the difference in average levels of red cell folate between the two groups has been less than 100 ng/ml. Our own figures show a difference of 50 ng/ml. This implies that a factor other than the drug is controlling red cell levels in both groups. Indeed, this is true, and we have found in our own studies that whether one is considering OC users or control subjects, the red cell folate level is very highly correlated with folacin intake. If folacin intake is low among a population of women receiving OC, then their red cell folate levels may be reduced to depletion levels, and such evidence as we have would suggest that they are at risk for the development of megaloblastic anemia. However, this last point should be accepted cautiously since conclusive proof is lacking. In determining which women are at risk I believe that we should be concerned with the folate status of the total population involved as reflected by the incidence of biochemical and hematological indices of folate deficiency in the total group.

Fisch and Friedman (15) showed that contraceptive steroids could produce changes in red cell parameters. In their population of middle-income women the blood changes brought about by use of OC were of minor extent and included a reduction in the red blood cell count and an elevation in the average mean corpuscular volume. In our own studies of the much lower income group of women, we have found a small but significant reduction in the erythrocyte count and significant elevation in mean corpuscular volume in the OC users. In our study, alcohol intake, as obtained by recall, was quantitatively related to average mean corpuscular volume, and the effects of alcohol and OC on this red cell index were additive but synergistic (16). It is suggested, then, that in the alcoholic woman whose folate status is precarious, intake of OC might be an added factor conducive to the development of megaloblastic anemia.

The actual number of published cases of megaloblastic anemia occurring among OC users has been 29, though other cases have been mentioned in the literature and we have observed one such case in a young woman on marginal intake of folacin (10, 12, 17–28). As indicated earlier, several of the women who have developed megaloblastic anemia while taking these drugs have subsequently been found to have malabsorption syndromes including overt or latent celiac disease.

Based on our own recent studies, which have shown that both in women taking OC and in those who are not taking these drugs erythrocyte folate values are closely correlated with intakes of dietary folacin, we have concluded that the risk of serious folate depletion developing in OC users is related largely to concurrent dietary folacin depletion, to alcoholism, and to the presence of malabsorption syndromes or other conditions, including usage of anticonvulsant drugs, in which folacin requirements are elevated (29). We would indeed concur with the finding of Kahn and co-workers (30) in pregnant women that the overall dietary intake of folate is the most important factor in the maintenance of adequate folate nutrition. Among healthy female undergraduates dietary factors that are associated with high levels of serum and red cell folate include intake of folic acid in breakfast cereals and intake of folic acid supplements. On the basis of estimates of erythrocyte folacin we have calculated that if the difference between OC and control groups is 50 ng/ml, then the increase in folic acid intake needed to compensate for this difference is 35 μg folic acid/day. It would appear that whereas quite small supplements of the vitamin would serve as a prophylaxis against folacin deficiency, higher supplementation would be required to overcome depletion. Because some women taking OC over a long period of time have already reached a state of moderate depletion, we would advocate that they receive a daily supplement on the order of 100 μg/day as folic acid (Kelley and Roe, unpublished). Inherent in the suggestion that a folic acid supplement or a fortified food equivalent should be advocated for use by women on OC is the belief that change in dietary habits to afford a higher intake of natural food folacin is more difficult to achieve.

Let us consider the significance of other changes in vitamin and mineral status that have been observed in women taking OC. Several authors have demonstrated that these drugs induce a lowering of serum vitamin B_{12} levels (31, 32). Evidence has been presented that whereas vitamin B_{12} absorption is normal in women taking these drugs, the rate of metabolism of the vitamin may be increased (33, 34). In a study of baboons carried out by Boots and associates (35), it was shown that whereas contraceptive steroids reduced serum levels of vitamin B_{12}, such levels were elevated by administration of pyridoxine. No explanation has been offered for this effect.

There have been several references in the literature to some impairment in riboflavin status associated with contraceptive steroid intake. The most important of these studies is that of Ahmed and associates (36), who investigated a group of Indian women whose diets were marginal in a number of nutrients. They found that riboflavin status was marginal in the women before OC and that after they took these drugs further evidence of riboflavin depletion appeared and some women developed glossitis. This study supports a general opinion that previous dietary inadequacy determines the adverse nutritional effects of OC.

A number of authors have shown that contraceptive steroids disturb tryptophan metabolism and there is evidence that this effect is dependent directly or indirectly on changes in vitamin B_6 status (37). Alterations in tryptophan metabolism associated with intake of contraceptive steroids are demonstrated by tryptophan load tests in which there is an increased excretion of xanthurenic acid and other metabolites in the tryptophan–nicotinic acid ribonucleotide pathway. These changes in tryptophan metabolism are reversed by administration of pyridoxine. It is apparently the estrogen component of contraceptive steroids that affects tryptophan metabolism, but the specific progestogen present in any particular combined OC may influence the degree of abnormality (38). It has further been suggested that depression occuring in women taking these drugs may be due to a relative vitamin B_6 deficiency since symptoms may be alleviated by administration of this vitamin (39). Whereas these and other reports, particularly by Rose's group, have suggested that OC users are vitamin B_6 dependent, we have been reassured by the studies of Lumeng et al. (40) that many women who continue to take OC for a period of time may adapt to altered pyridoxine utilization. They found that although significant decreases in plasma pyridoxal phosphate occurred after contraceptive steroid intake began, there tended to be a return to pre-treatment levels in most subjects by the sixth month of treatment.

Evidence of mild thiamic depletion has been presented by Briggs and Briggs (41). Changes in thiamine status as reflected by biochemical tests including erythrocyte transketolase activity were also found in OC users by Ahmed and co-workers (36), but these authors have cautioned us against accepting without further study that these findings represent a state of hypovitaminosis.

Several authors have shown that ascorbic acid levels in plasma, leukocytes, and platelets are reduced by contraceptive steroids. It has also been demonstrated that the estrogenic component of these agents is responsible for this effect (42–45). Rivers has viewed the literature on this subject and has noted that increases in plasma levels of ascorbic acid after administration of vitamin C supplements are less in OC users than in control subjects. She has further suggested that the effects of OC on vitamin C levels reflect alteration in distribution of the vitamin, particularly tissue distribution (46).

Regardless of the socioeconomic status or other demographic characteristics of the women studied, a common finding has been elevated plasma vitamin A levels. This was first observed by Gal and co-workers in 1971 (47). It has therefore been suggested that women receiving OC may have a decreased requirement for vitamin A (48). There was some concern that these high vitamin A levels could constitute a teratogenic hazard if a woman became pregnant soon after discontinuing the pill. However, in a study by Wilde and associates (49), it was shown that during early pregnancy there was no significant difference in vitamin A levels between women who had recently taken OC and those who had not.

A number of studies have attempted to clarify the risk of thromboembolic phenomena occurring as a side effect of OC intake (50, 51). The risk of thromboses is related to the estrogen content of the OC (52). In the laboratory rat, estrogens diminish the requirement for vitamin K (53). Increased serum levels of vitamin K-dependent clotting factors as well as other clotting factors have been found in women taking OC (54–56). Mink and co-workers (57) monitored the effects of sequential OC on serum clotting factors in a group of women under observation for two years. Vitamin K-dependent factor activity was elevated in women after three months of taking OC, and remained elevated for the period of study. These observations suggest that the need for vitamin K is reduced by OC. In further support of this theory, it has been shown that women taking OC exhibit a subnormal response to coumarin anticoagulants (58).

Plasma vitamin E levels may be slightly raised in women taking OC, an effect noted only in humans which may be related to changes in lipoprotein distribution rather than altered nutritional status. In rats, plasma vitamin E levels are reduced by administration of combined estrogen (mestranol) and progestogen (norethynodrel) (59, 60).

Iron is a nutrient for which OC users may have a smaller demand. Women taking OC tend to have a reduced menstrual blood loss and hence reduced iron loss. Further, it has been shown that serum iron levels as well as total iron-binding capacity may be elevated concomitantly in women taking OC

(61, 62). In studies of our own student population we have not found significant differences in serum iron levels between OC users and control subjects, though we have found the previously described changes in total iron-binding capacity. We attribute this to differences in iron intake according to dietary level and level of supplementation, both in our contraceptive drug users and in the remaining students (Halstead and Roe, unpublished).

In OC users changes have been found in the plasma levels of copper and zinc, the former being elevated and the latter depressed. It is generally considered that the elevations in plasma copper are mainly due to elevated levels of ceruloplasmin, which also occurs in OC users (63). Increased synthesis and levels of mineral-binding proteins including ceruloplasmin and transferrin are estrogen-induced effects (64). Decreased plasma levels of zinc were reported first by Halsted and co-workers, and subsequently by a number of other authors (65, 66). Prasad and associates found, as did these other authors that plasma zinc levels were depressed by OC use but that there was an associated increase in erythrocyte zinc levels. They have suggested the possibility that there is a redistribution of zinc induced by OC because of enhanced binding of this mineral in the red cells to the apoenzyme of carbonic anhydrase, a protein which may be induced by OC (62). The nutritional aberrations that have been corrected with the use of contraceptive steroids are summarized in Table 1.

Table 1 Nutritional Aberrations Attributed to Contraceptive Steroids

Nutrient	Effect
Folacin	Serum level decreased
	Erythrocyte level decreased
	Megaloblastic anemia (rare)
Vitamin B_{12}	Serum level decreased
Riboflavin	Erythrocyte level decreased
	Glossitis (rare)
Vitamin B_6	Disturbed tryptophan metabolism
	Plasma PLP decreased
	Depression
Ascorbic acid	Leukocyte content decreased
	Platelet level decreased
Vitamin A	Plasma level increased
Iron	Serum level increased
	TIBC increased
Copper	Plasma copper increased
	Ceruloplasmin increased
Zinc	Plasma zinc decreased

NUTRITIONAL INTERVENTION AND CONTRACEPTIVE STEROID USAGE

With the bewildering array of information on the nutritional effects of these drugs, we are left with the question whether we should intervene to reverse the observed changes. Whether women taking OC need supplementary vitamins and perhaps minerals must depend largely on their accustomed diet and other major factors that determine their nutritional status. We need to know more about the effects of these drugs on the nutritional status of very high risk groups such as girls in the early adolescent period for whom oral contraceptives are now being prescribed. We need to know more about the nutritional status of women on these drugs in parts of the world where the prevailing diet is marginal or deficient, particularly in one or more B vitamins. We need to know why these nutritional changes occur, and what is their significance. However, I believe that even now we have enough data to make some public policy. We may wish to consider the route we may take. There is much to be said in favor of staple food supplementation and there is already a trend in this direction in this country, where a number of breakfast foods including breakfast cereals have been fortified not only with the usual range of vitamins and minerals, but also with folic acid. We have demonstrated the effectiveness of these cereals in overcoming folate depletion among some of the OC users whom we have studied. Providing these fortified foods is a useful measure but it seems unlikely that they will be eaten by those most at risk, because of cost, ingrown food habits, and lack of availability outside the United States.

Another suggestion is that we provide nutrient supplements specifically formulated to the needs of OC users. There are now a number of vitamin preparations being marketed which contain folic acid at a level supplying 100 μg/day which would be appropriate to the needs of women taking OC. However, most of these vitamin pills contain vitamin A, and we believe that this is neither necessary nor useful. Indeed, in young women who consume large amounts of vitamin A in the diet, it could conceivably be hazardous. Finally we can consider the addition of specific vitamins to OC pills. The argument here is which vitamins to add. My prejudice is for folic acid, and possibly pyridoxine. Before we can seriously advocate the large-scale use of any of these measures it will be necessary to compare one method with another. Meanwhile, I would like to offer a few words of caution. The nutritional problems of women who take these drugs are small compared to the problems that result from inadequate diets or repeated pregnancies. Nutritional problems should be recognized, but not exaggerated, and where possible they should be avoided by knowing the risks and by giving the appropriate nutritional advice.

Finally we should realize that from the nutritional standpoint there are women for whom long-term administration of these drugs is contraindicated and for whom alternative methods of contraception would be more appropriate.

REFERENCES

1. Klopper, A. Developments in steroidal hormonal contraception. *Brit. Med. Bull.* **26**:39 (1970).
2. Population Report 1974. Oral contraceptives—fifty million users. Series A, No. 1, Dept. Medicine and Public Affairs, George Washington University Medical Center, Washington, D.C.
3. American Medical Association Drug Evaluations, 2nd ed. Publishing Sciences Group, Acton, Mass., 1973, p. 411.
4. Briggs, M. H., Pitchford, A. G., Staniford, M., Barker, H. M., and Taylor, D. Metabolic effects of steroid contraceptive. In *Advances in Steroid Biochemistry and Pharmacology*. M. H. Briggs, Ed. Vol. 2, Academic, London and New York, 1970, p. 111.
5. Doll, R., and Vessey, M. P. Evaluation of rare adverse effects of systemic contraceptives. *Brit. Med. Bull.* **56**:33 (1970).
6. Bakker, C. B., and Dightman, C. R. Side effects of oral contraceptives. *Obstet. Gynecol.* **28**:373 (1966).
7. Roe, D. A. and Eickwort, K. R. Health and nutritional status of working and non-working mothers in poverty groups. Research Contract No. 51–36–71–02, Manpower Administration, U.S.D.L., 1973.
8. Shojania, A. M., Hornady, G., and Barnes, P. H. Oral contraceptives and serum folate levels. *Lancet* **1**:1376 (1968).
9. Shojania, A. M., Hornady, G., and Barnes, P. H. Oral contraceptives and folate metabolism. *Lancet* **1**:886 (1969).
10. Shojania, A. M., and Hornady, G. J. Oral contraceptives and folate absorption. *J. Lab. Clin. Med.* **82**:869 (1971).
11. Shojania, A. M. The effect of oral contraceptives on folate metabolism. III. Plasma clearance and urinary folate excretion. *J. Lab. Clin. Med.* **85**:185 (1975).
12. Streiff, R. R. Folate deficiency and oral contraceptives *J.A.M.A.* **214**:105 (1970).
13. Stephens, M. E. M., Craft, I., Peters, T. J., and Hoffbrand, A. V. Oral contraceptives and folate metabolism *Clin. Sci.* **42**:405 (1972).
14. Martinez, O. and Roe, D. A. Diet and contraceptive steroids (OCA) as determinants of folate status in pregnancy. *Fed. Proc.* **33**:715 (1974).
15. Fisch, I. R., and Friedman, S. H. Oral contraceptives and the red blood cell. *Clin. Pharm. Therap.* **14**:245 (1973).
16. Roe, D. A. Drug, diet and diagnostic criteria as determinants of the folate status of women on oral contraceptives. Presented at Proc. 10th Internat. Congr. Nutr., Kyoto, Japan, Aug. 3–9, 1975.
17. Paton, A. Oral contraceptives and folate deficiency. *Lancet* **1**:418 (1969).

18. Necheles, T. F., and Snyder, L. M. Malabsorption of folate polyglutamates associated with oral contraceptive therapy. *New Engl. J. Med.* **282**:858 (1970).

19. Holmes, R. P. Megaloblastic anemia precipitated by the use of oral contraceptives. *N. Carolina Med. J.* **31**:17 (1970).

20. Toghill, P. J., and Smith, P. G. Folate deficiency and the pill. Brit. Med. J. **1**:608 (1971).

21. Buhac, I., and Finn, J. W. Folsauremangelanamie als Folge des langfristigen Gebrauchs peroraler kontranzeptiver Mittel. *Schweiz. Med. Wochschr.* **101**:1879 (1971).

22. Palva, P. Megaloblastisk anemia orsaked av orala kontraseptiva. *Nord. Med.* **86**:1491 (1971).

23. Ryser, J. E., Farquet, J. J., and Petite, J. Megaloblastic anemia due to folic acid deficiency in a young woman on oral contraceptives. *Acta Haematol.* **45**:319 (1971).

24. Wood, J. K., Goldstone, A. H., and Allan, N. C. Folic acid and the pill. *Scand. J. Haematol.* **9**:539 (1972).

25. Salter, W. M. Megaloblastic anemia and oral contraceptives. *Minn. Med.* **55**:554 (1972).

26. Flury, R., and Angehrn, W. Folsauremangelanamie infolge Einnahme oraler Kontrazeptiva. *Schweiz. Med. Wochschr.* **102**:1628 (1972).

27. Johnson, G. K., Greene, J. E., Hensley, G. T., and Soergel, K. H. Small intestinal disease, folate deficiency anemia, and oral contraceptive agents. *Am. J. Digest. Dis.* **18**:253 (1973).

28. Alperin, J. B. Folate metabolism in women using oral contraceptive agents. *Am. J. Clin. Nutr.* **26**:xix (1973) (abst.).

29. Roe, D. A. Effects of drugs on nutrition. *Life Sci.* **15**:1219 (1974).

30. Kahn, S. B., Fein, S., Rigberg, S., and Brodsky, I. Correlation of folate metabolism and socioeconomic status in pregnancy and in patients taking oral contraceptives. *Am. J. Obstet. Gynecol.* **108**:931 (1970).

31. Briggs, M. H., and Briggs, M. Oral contraceptives and vitamin nutrition. *Lancet* **1**:1234 (1974).

32. Smith, J. L., Goldsmith, G. A., and Lawrence, J. D. Effects of oral contraceptive steroids on vitamin and lipid levels in serum. *Am. J. Clin. Nutr.* **28**:371 (1975).

33. Shojania, A. M. Effect of oral contraceptives on vitamin B_{12} metabolism. *Lancet* **2**:932 (1971).

34. Wertalik, L. F., Metz, E. M., LoBuglio, A. F., and Balcerzak, S. P. Decreased serum B_{12} levels with oral contraceptive use. *J.A.M.A.* **21**:1371 (1972).

35. Boots, L., Cornwell, P. E., and Beck, L. R. Effect of ethynodiol diacetate and mestranol on serum folic acid and vitamin B_{12} levels and on tryptophan metabolism in baboons. *Am. J. Clin. Nutr.* **28**:54 (1975).

36. Ahmed, F., Bamjo, M. S., and Iyengar, L. Effect of oral contraceptive agents on vitamin nutrition status. *Am. J. Clin. Nutr.* **28**:606 (1975).

37. Price, J. M., Thornton, M. J., and Mueller, L. M. Tryptophan metabolism in women using steroid hormones for ovulation control. *Am. J. Clin. Nutr.* **20**:452 (1967).

38. Rose, D. P., Adams, P. W., and Strong, R. Influence of the progestogenic com-

ponents of oral contraceptives on tryptophan metabolism. *J. Obstet. Gynecol.* **80**:82 (1973).

39. Adams, P. W., Rose, D. P., Folkar, D. J., Wynn, V., Seed, M., and Strong, R. Effect of pyridoxine hydrochloride (vitamin B_6) upon depression associated with oral contraception. *Lancet* **1**:897 (1973).
40. Lumeng L., Cleary, R. E., and Li, P-K. Effect of oral contraceptives on the plasma concentration of pyridoxal phosphate. *Am. J. Clin. Nutr.* **27**:326 (1974).
41. Briggs, M. H., and Briggs, M. Thiamine status and oral contraceptives. *Contraception* **11**:151 (1975).
42. Rivers, J. M., and Devine, M. M. Plasma ascorbic acid concentrations and oral contraceptives. *Am. J. Clin. Nutr.* **25**:684 (1972).
43. McLeroy, V. J., and Schendel, H. E. Influence of oral contraceptives on ascorbic acid concentrations in healthy, sexually mature women. *Am. J. Clin. Nutr.* **26**:191 (1973).
44. Briggs, M. H., and Briggs, M. Vitamin C requirements and oral contraceptives. *Nature* **238**:277 (1972).
45. Kalesh, B. G., Mallikarjuneswara, V. R., and Clemetson, C. A. B. Effect of estrogen containing oral contraceptives on platelet and plasma ascorbic acid concentrations. *Contraception* **4**:183 (1971).
46. Rivers, J .M. Oral contraceptives and ascorbic acid. *Am. J. Clin. Nutr.* **28**:550 (1975).
47. Gal. L., Parkinson, C., and Kraft, I. Effect of oral contraceptives on human plasma vitamin A levels. *Brit. Med. J.* **2**:436 (1971).
48. Theuer, R. C. Effect of oral contraceptive agents on vitamin and mineral needs: A review. *J. Repro. Med.* **8**:13 (1972).
49. Wilde, J., Schorah, C. H., and Smithells, W. Vitamin A, pregnancy and oral contraceptives. *Brit. Med. J.* **1**:57 (1974).
50. Vessey, M. P., and Doll, R. Investigations of relation between use of oral contraceptives and thromboembolic disease. *Brit. Med. J.* 2:199 (1968).
51. Vessey, M. P., and Doll, R. Investigation of relation between use of oral contraceptives and thromboembolic disease. A further report. *Brit. Med. J.* **2**:651 (1969).
52. Inman, W. H. W., Vessey, M. P., Westerholm, B., and Engelund, A. Thromboembolic disease and the steroidal content of oral contraceptives. A report to the committee on safety of drugs. *Brit. Med. J.* **2**:203 (1970).
53. Mellette, S. J. Interrelationships between vitamin K and estrogenic hormones. *Am. J. Clin. Nutr.* **9**, suppl., 109 (1961).
54. Egeberge, O., and Owren, P. A. Contraception and blood coagulability. *Brit. Med. J.* **1**:220 (1963).
55. Rutherford, R. N., Hougie, C., Bankes, A. L., and Coburn, W. A. The effects of sex steroids and pregnancy on blood coagulation factors. Comparative study. *Obstet Gynecol.* **24**:886 (1964).
56. D'Arcy, P. F., and Griffin, J. P. *Iatrogenic Diseases.* Oxford, New York, 1972, p. 57.
57. Mink, I. B., Conney, N. G., Niswander, K. R., et al. Progestational agents and blood coagulation. V. Changes induced by sequential oral contraceptive therapy. *Am. J. Obstet. Gynecol.* **119**:401 (1974).

58. Scrogie, J. J., Solomon, H. M., and Zieve, P. D. Effect of oral contraceptives on vitamin K-dependent clotting activity. *Clin. Pharmacol. Therap.* **8**:670 (1967).
59. Yeung, D. L. and Chan, P. L. Effects of a progestogen and a sequential type oral contraceptive on plasma vitamin A, vitamin E, cholesterol and triglycerides. *Am. J. Clin. Nutr.* **28**:686 (1975).
60. Aftergood, L. and Alfin-Slater, R. B. Oral contraceptive-α tocopherol interrelationships. *Lipids* **9**:91 (1974).
61. Mardell, M., Symmons, C., and Zilva, J. F. A comparison of the effect of oral contraceptives, pregnancy and sex on iron metabolism. *J. Clin. Endocrinol.* **29**:1489 (1969).
62. Prasad, A. S., Oberleas, D., Lei, K. Y., Moghissi, K. S., and Stryker, J. C. Effect of oral contraceptive agents on nutrients: I. Minerals. *Am. J. Clin. Nutr.* **28**:377 (1975).
63. Carruthers, M. E., Hobbs, C. B., and Warren, R. L. Raised serum copper and ceruloplasmin levels in subjects taking oral contraceptives. *J. Clin. Pathol.* **19**:498 (1966).
64. Briggs, M. H., and Briggs, M. Contraceptives and serum proteins. *Brit. Med. J.* **3**:521 (1970).
65. Halsted, J. A., Hackley, B. M., and Smith, Jr., J. C. Plasma, zinc and copper in pregnancy and after oral contraceptives. *Lancet* **2**:278 (1968).
66. O'Leary, J. A., and Spellacy, W. N. Zinc and copper levels in pregnant women and those taking oral contraceptives. *Am. J. Obstet. Gynecol.* **102**:131 (1969).

PART 2

Nutrition during Different Periods of Life

4

Factors that Affect Nutritional Requirements in Adolescents

JO ANNE BRASEL, M.D.

Institute of Human Nutrition, College of Physicians and Surgeons, Columbia University, New York, New York

Adolescence is a period of great turmoil and change. Psychologically the adolescent is striving toward the independence of adulthood while remaining dependent financially and emotionally on parents. Wide swings in mood and temperament and demanding and inconsistent behavior often tax the patience of the adults in the immediate environment. Decisions regarding career choice and relationships with the opposite sex must be made in the face of societal constraints that often conflict with the degree of physiological maturation. Physically the adolescent male has the muscle strength to perform many occupational tasks reserved for adults, and both sexes become sexually mature and capable of procreation long before this is acceptable in today's western society. Peer pressures and acceptance become all-important and often run counter to parental expectations. No wonder, then, that most parents of teenagers and many physicians who deal with adolescents have come to think of adolescence as a medical and psychiatric disorder, characterized by rage fits, rebellion, excessive growth of scalp and facial hair, and disturbances in eating patterns, interspersed with paroxysms of normal behavior.

The changes in growth are equally striking. Body weight is nearly doubled during the adolescent growth spurt, and approximately 15% is added toward adult height. This chapter will focus on the changes that occur in body growth and composition during adolescence. Although this book is concerned principally with the female, it is nearly impossible to discuss the female's adolescence without comparing it to the male's, and therefore changes noted in both sexes will be described. Finally we shall attempt to translate the composition of the growth into nutritional requirements.

Adolescence, as seen physically in terms of sexual development, is the result of the secretion of the sex hormones: testosterone produced by the Leydig cells of the testes and estrogens produced by the developing Graafian follicles of the ovaries. Androgens produced by the adrenal cortex may also play some role in adolescent development, especially in the female. The increased secretion of these hormones occurs in response to stimulation of the gonads by the gonadotropic hormones, LH and FSH, which in turn are released following hormonal stimulation of the anterior pituitary by the gonadotropin-releasing factors of the hypothalamus. The control of the initiation of puberty is largely a mystery, but as we shall see later, it may have some relationship to reaching a "critical" body weight or state of skeletal development that in some manner sets off the "adolescent alarm clock." Once established, the mature hypothalamic-pituitary-gonadal axis operates in a finely tuned fashion to cause cyclic release of ova in the female and continuous sperm formation in the male until the gonodal failure of senescence occurs. The secretion of increased amounts of sex hormones at adolescence is responsible not only for sexual development, but also for the growth spurt and the changes in body composition that occur at this time of life, since subjects without functional ovaries or testes do not experience a growth spurt and continue to have a prepubertal or "neuter" body composition in adult life.

What are the changes in physical appearance and sexual development which lead to an adult body configuration and reproductive capacity? Tanner and his co-workers have examined a number of normal children longitudinally and divided pubertal development into five stages beginning with Stage 1, the prepubertal child, and ending with Stage 5, full adult sexual development.

Breast development in the female progresses as shown in Fig. 1 and may be described as follows:

Stage 1. No palpable glandular tissue. Areola is not pigmented. Except for nipple, breast does not project from anterior chest wall.

Stage 2. Glandular tissue is palpable, at least as a nubbin underneath the areola. Nipple and breast project as a single mound from the chest wall.

Stage 3. Glandular tissue is further increased in size. Areola increases in diameter and becomes pigmented, but contour of breast and Areola remain in a single plane of projection.

Stage 4. Further enlargement of glandular tissue is noted. Areola is more darkly pigmented. Areola and nipple form a secondary mound above the level of the breast.

Stage 5 (Maturity). Areola and nipple no longer form a separate mound but

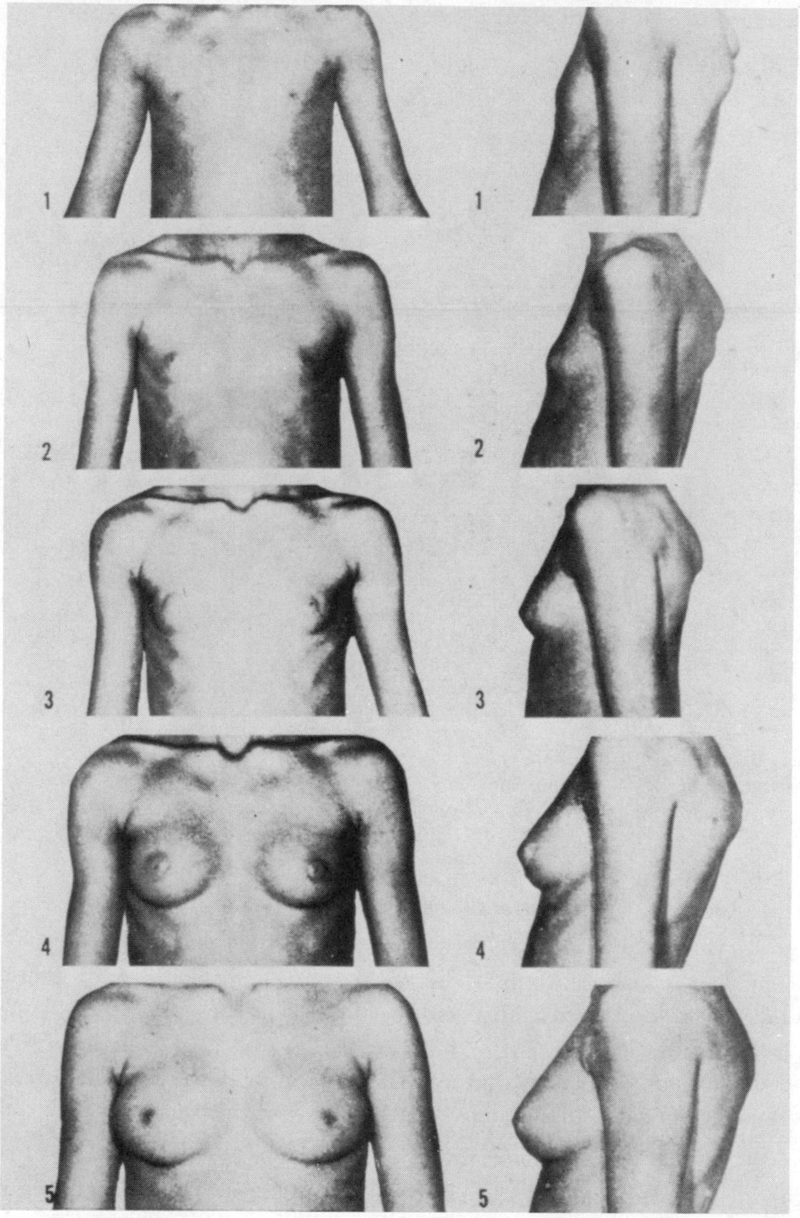

Figure 1. Breast development in the female. Reproduced with kind permission from Tanner, J. M., Growth and Endocrinology of the Adolescent. In *Endocrine and Genetic Diseases of Childhood*. Saunders, Philadelphia, 1969.

recede to make a smooth contour in profile view. In some women this stage is never reached or does not occur until after a pregnancy.

The stages of pubic hair development in the female are shown in Fig. 2 and may be decribed as follows:

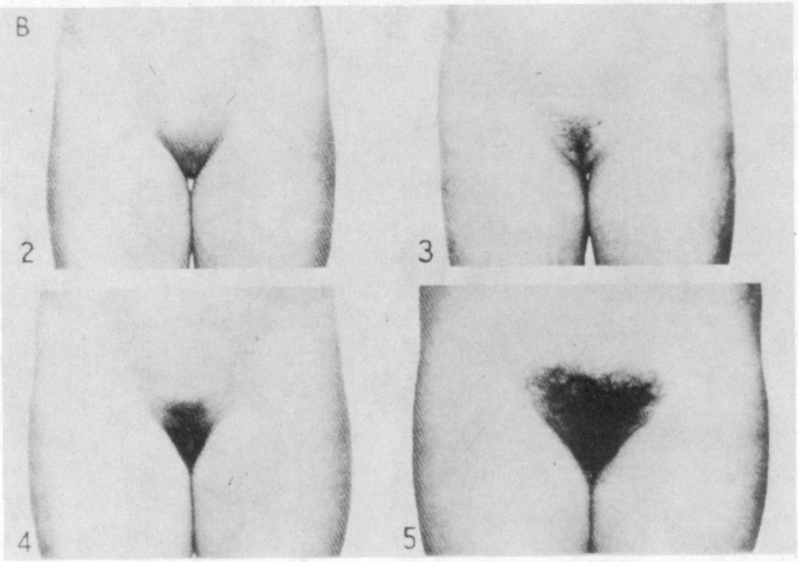

Figure 2. Pubic hair development in the female. Reproduced with kind permission of the author and publisher from Tanner, J. M., Growth and Endocrinology of the Adolescent. In *Endocrine and Genetic Diseases of Childhood*, Saunders, Philadelphia, 1969.

Stage 1. None.

Stage 2. Occasional wispy strands, usually along the labia majora.

Stage 3. More, darker, and coarser hair extends superiorly over the pubis.

Stage 4. Dark, coarse curly hair covers the mons pubis in the adult pattern, but does not extend to the medial aspects of the thighs.

Stage 5. Mature state in which hair extends to the medial aspects of the thighs; in a small percentage of normal women hair extends varying distances above the mons pubis in a diamond pattern toward the umbilicus in a "male like" pattern.

Breast changes usually are the first signs of puberty to appear and require approximately four years to complete. Pubic hair usually appears later but takes less time—approximately three years—to reach Stage 5. Axillary hair usually appears when breasts are in Stage 3 or 4. By the time the average girl has reached Stage 3 of breast development and pubic hair growths, she is at the peak of her growth spurt in height and weight. Although menarche, i.e., the first menstrual period, can occur during Stage 2, it is Stage 4 before 85 to 90% of girls reach menarche. The beginning of menses heralds a rapid decline in growth rate and most girls grow less than a total of two inches after their first menstrual period. Cyclic ovulation and regular menses normally are seen within two years of menarche.

Although the timing of pubertal development is influenced by genetic background, other factors are of equal, if not greater, importance. Social class, urban vs. rural environment, and altitude may all play a role. However, when these factors are examined closely, their common denominator seems to be effect on growth rate, since larger girls enter puberty earlier than smaller ones. The level of general health and nutritional status are undoubtedly very important in this regard. It is now well known that during the past 100 to 125 years the mean age of menarche has decreased at a rate of 3 to 4 months per decade and now appears to be leveling off in western Europe and in the United States. Although the mean age at menarche has declined from 17.0 to 13.0 years, the mean weight at menarche (47 kg) has not changed. This has led Frisch and co-workers to postulate a "critical mass" hypothesis, stating that the initiation of the growth spurt, the time of peak growth velocity, and menarches occur at certain "invariant" weights, regardless of the chronological age of the subject. Epidemiological data would certainly support this hypothesis. However in examining normal girls in good health in the developed world, there are certainly exceptions to this theory, so that the earlier statement that the control of the initiation of pubery is largely a mystery remains justified. On the average, in normal girls the initiation of the growth spurt in height begins at 9.6 years, Stage 2 peak height velocity is reached at 11.8 years, breast development is seen at 11.2 years, and menarche occurs at 12.5 years. There are normal variations about these means, as for any biological phenomena, which must be taken into account when assessing adolescent development in any one subject. However, any girl who menstruates before age 9 or after age 16 should be considered outside the range of normal.

The adolescent development of the male genitalia has also been described in stages by Tanner and is shown in Fig. 3.

Stage 1. The prepubertal stage persists from birth until puberty begins. The genitalia appear infantile and change very little during this stage except to grow somewhat in overall size along with the rest of the body.

Stage 2. The first evidence of puberty is characterized by enlargement of the testes and scrotum along with some reddening and thinning of the scrotal skin.

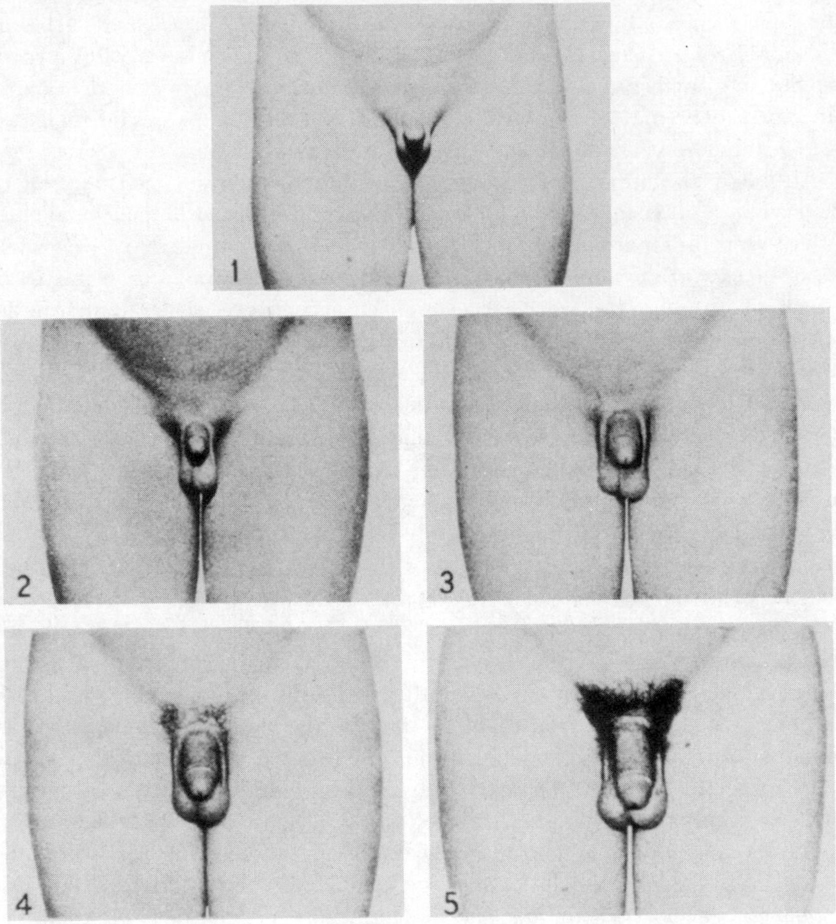

Figure 3. Pubic hair and genital development in the male. Reproduced with kind permission of the author and publisher from Tanner, J. M., Growth and Endocrinology of the Adolescent. In *Endocrine and Genetic Diseases of Childhood*, Saunders, Philadelphia, 1969.

Stage 3. The phallus increases in length and to a small extent in breadth. The testes and scrotum continue to enlarge.

Stage 4. The phallus increases further in length and breadth. The glans becomes developed. The testes and scrotum are larger and scrotal skin is becoming darkly pigmented.

Stage 5. The genitalia are adult in size and shape.

The development of pubic hair in boys can be divided into five stages using criteria similar to those for girls. In most men sexual hair spreads up the abdomen in a diamond-shaped pattern, but this is seldom achieved before age 20 and, therefore, is usually not considered a part of pubertal development. Recession of the hair line in the temporal regions in males is not noted until middle to late adolescence. Axillary hair is not usually seen until development of the genitalia is well advanced and is usually noted one to two years later than pubic hair. The first sign of facial hair growth is an increase in the length and pigmentation of hairs at the corner of the upper lip. The mustache is usually complete before much hair grows on the upper part of the cheek. Beard growth over the lower jaw and chin is the last to appear.

The voice deepens as the larynx enlarges, which occurs in late puberty. The prostate gland enlarges under the influence of testosterone and becomes easily palpable on rectal exam during middle to late puberty. There is frequently some glandular enlargement of the breast during the male adolescence, which is ordinarily self-limited and regresses on its own; it is most common in those boys with the most rapid virilization who presumably have the highest male hormone levels.

An increase in testis size, the first sign of beginning pubertal development in boys, is unusually early if noted before 9.5 years and late if not present by 13.7 years. The mean age of reaching Stage 2 is 11.6 years. The average boy will have completed genital development by 14.9 years, but it may occur as early as 12.7 or as late as 17.1 years. The progression from one stage to the next is quite variable, and one boy may take as long to progress from Stage 2 to 3 as another takes to complete the whole process. About 75% of normal males reach peak height and weight velocity while in Stage 4 of genital development and only 2% reach peak velocity before that time. Therefore boys who are concerned about their height and have not yet reached Stage 4 of development can be reassured that their growth spurt is yet to come. The mean age of peak height velocity for males is 14 years, approximately two years later than that for females.

What changes in hormone secretion are responsible for the sexual development? In the female small increases in serum LH and FSH are noted between 6 and 10 years of age, but estradiol levels do not change before age 10. The earliest signs of puberty, the appearance of a subareolar breast bud or labial hair, are accompanied by elevations in serum FSH and estradiol. Serum LH levels increase significantly above the prepubertal values in midpuberty when secondary sexual characteristics are well developed. After menarche adult levels of estradiol are achieved and serum LH and FSH demonstrate a wide scatter in values due to fluctuations occurring within the menstrual cycle. Progesterone becomes measurable once ovulation occurs. This pattern of hormone release confirms and extends earlier work which led to naming one gonadotropin follicle-stimulating hormone (FSH), because of its effects on the Graafiian follicle leading to estrogen production, and to naming the other luteinizing hormone (LH), which produces other effects on the follicle, ultimately leading to ovulation and subsequently to progesterone production.

In the male gradual increases in serum LH and FSH and in testicle size occur between the ages of 6 and 10 years. The earliest recognizable pubertal change, the increase in testis growth, is accompanied by continued increases in FSH, which begins to rise before LH and reaches adult levels of approximately twice the prepubertal values before either LH or testosterone. After age 12, a significant increment in the rise of serum LH is noted and is accompanied by significant increases in serum testosterone levels. Testosterone levels increase approximately twentyfold between 10 and 17 years of age, while LH shows a threefold increase between childhood and adulthood. The more marked increases in both LH and testosterone occur between 12 and 14 years in the average boy. This pattern of hormone release supports a model in which LH plays a primary role in Leydig cell development and testosterone secretion, while FSH plays a role in testicular growth and siminiferous tubular development, including sperm formation.

What are the dimensions of the adolescent growth spurt? What is the composition of the added tissue and how do the sexes differ? The rapid weight gain characteristic of the immediate postnatal months decreases to an average of 2 to 3 kg/year during the mid-childhood years, with little difference between the sexes until girls enter their adolescent spurt followed two years later by boys. At peak velocity the average girl gains 8.3 kg/year, with a range of 5.5 kg for the 3rd percentile girl to 10.6 for the 97th percentile girl. The mean peak velocity for boys is 9.0 kg, with ranges from 6.1 to 12.8 kg/year.

There is little difference in yearly height gains between the sexes before girls enter adolescence. The 50th percentile for peak height velocity in girls is 8.3 cm, with ranges of 6.2 to 10.4 cm/year. The corresponding figures for boys are a mean peak of 9.4 cm, with ranges of 7.2 to 11.8 cm/year. Thus men are taller than women because they enter adolescence later and gain 5 to 6 cm in these two extra years of growth and because they grow more than girls during the adolescent spurt. In general, it also follows that children entering adolescence early tend to be shorter adults and those entering adolescence late taller, other factors being equal.

Studies of body composition changes during adolescence reveal distinct differences between the sexes. In general males deposit proportionately more lean body tissue and skeletal mass while females deposit proportionately more fat. The studies that lead to these conclusions have been performed on normal subjects by a number of investigators and include measurement of total body water, total body potassium, and total body fat.

In Fig. 4 total body water is plotted against height for normal males and

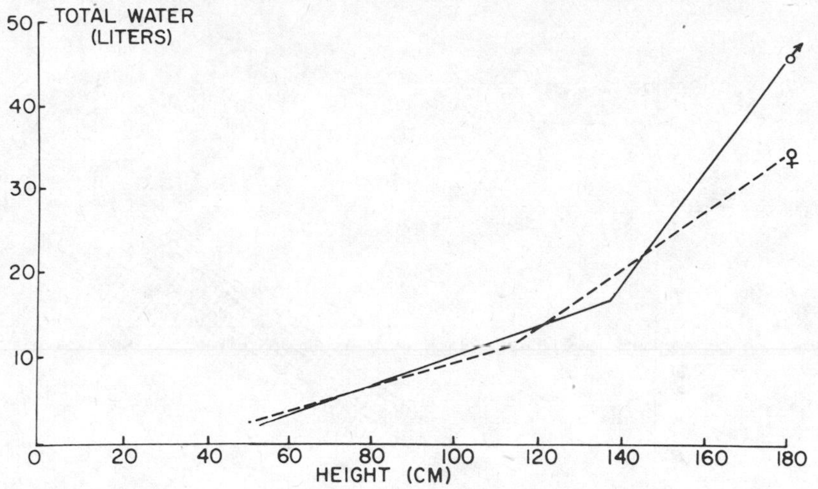

Figure 4. Total body water versus height in normal males and females. Reproduced with kind permission of author and publisher from Cheek, D. B., Body Composition, Hormones, Nutrition and Adolescent Growth. In *Control of the Onset of Puberty*, Wiley, New York, 1974.

females. Since the greatest proportion of body water resides within the cells and since fat tissue is anhydrous, total body water is an indirect measure of lean body mass. Additionally since the one greatest lean tissue mass is muscle, total body water reflects growth in skeletal muscle to a large extent. At a height of 130 to 140 cm in males the slope of the curve rises steeply, indicating an addition of greater amounts of lean tissue deposited for each centimeter in height gained thereafter. This change in slope occurs at 10 to 11 years of age, i.e., at the beginning of the adolescent growth spurt. Note that in females the change in slope is significantly less steep and that it occurs at 110 cm, reflecting the earlier onset of puberty.

Similar conclusions can be drawn from measurements of total body potassium, which, as a predominantly intracellular ion, is also a measure of lean body mass. The data of Flynn and co-workers, shown in Fig. 5, demonstrate that after girls reach approximately 130 to 140 cm in height, they deposit less potassium, and therefore less lean tissue, than boys for each centimeter gained. Forbes has converted his measurements of total body potassium to a ratio of lean body mass to height; a distinct divergence is noted at 13 years when the lean body mass gained per unit height increases over earlier childhood values in boys, and by contrast, begins to level off in girls.

If, on the other hand, body fat is measured during growth and development, boys can be shown to increase fat deposition during their adolescence, but the increase is modest and at 180 cm of height fat mass averages about

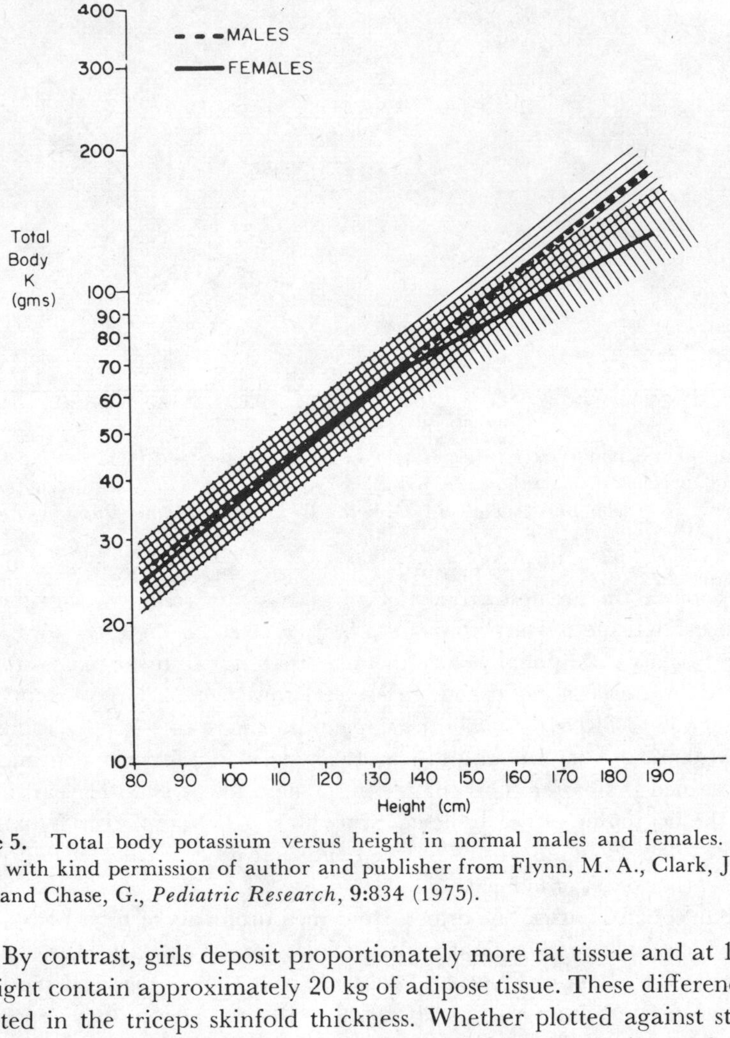

Figure 5. Total body potassium versus height in normal males and females. Reproduced with kind permission of author and publisher from Flynn, M. A., Clark, J., Reid, J. C., and Chase, G., *Pediatric Research*, 9:834 (1975).

9 kg. By contrast, girls deposit proportionately more fat tissue and at 180 cm in height contain approximately 20 kg of adipose tissue. These differences are reflected in the triceps skinfold thickness. Whether plotted against stage of puberty or chronological age, the thickness increases during puberty in females and actually decreases in males.

These various changes in growth and body composition, in terms of velocity, have recently been conveniently plotted by Barnes for both sexes on one graph (Fig. 6). The time of peak height velocities and age of menarches are shown by the vertical dashed lines. The greater muscle mass deposition in males and the greater fat deposition in females is readily apparent, as well as the time of peak growth in tissues in relation to peak height and weight gains.

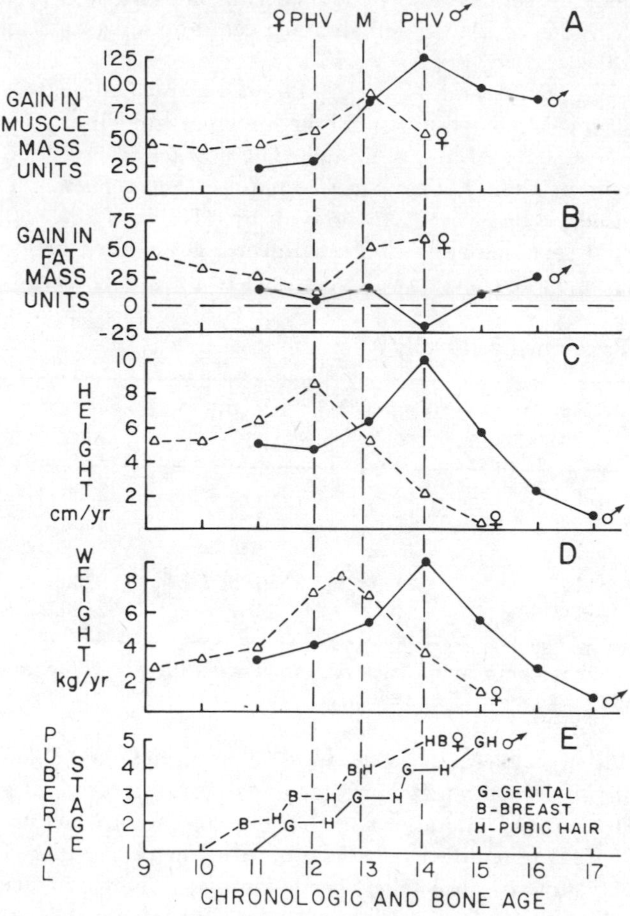

Figure 6. Composite figure of growth and compositional changes during adolescence. Reproduced with kind permission of author and publisher from Barnes, H. V., *Med. Clin. N. Am.*, **59**:1305 (1975).

How can these data be related to nutritional requirements? One might calculate the amount of protein, calories, and minerals required to build up the amounts of tissue deposited during adolescence, and add that to basal requirements, spreading the derived requirements out over the period of adolescence. Similar methods have been used in animal husbandry, but such calculations are unlikely to be of value in human populations. First, the requirements are greatest at the time of peak growth, which varies from subject to subject. Second, no consideration is made for activity, which has considerable influence on requirements and is likewise extremely variable. Third, even if reasonable and individual calculations could be made, what then? Have you ever tried to tell an adolescent anything, especially what he or she should eat?

In 1974 the Food and Nutrition Board of the National Academy of Sciences of the United States published revised guidelines of energy and protein requirements for all age groups. The portion covering the adolescent years is shown in Table 1. The suggested requirements reflect an increase over levels required for basal needs and growth by a factor of 20 to 30% to allow for individual variation above the usual needs. Hopefully, therefore, anyone meeting the suggested intakes will satisfy his or her needs with some leeway.

Table 1 Recommended Daily Allowances[a]

	Age (yr)	Weight (kg)	Height (cm)	Energy (kcal)	Protein (g)
Males	11–14	44	158	2800	44
	15–18	61	172	3000	54
Females	11–14	44	155	2400	44
	15–18	54	162	2100	48

[a] Adapted from Recommended Dietary Allowances, 8th ed., National Academy of Sciences, 1974.

In conclusion, adolescence is a period of unprecedented change and upheaval. Nutrition requirements are increased because of rapid growth and tissue deposition and alterations in the level of physical activity. Previous nutritional status may affect the initiation of adolescence through its effects on childhood growth, since taller, heavier subjects enter adolescence earlier than shorter, lighter ones. Failure to meet the nutritional needs at the time of adolescence may adversely affect the process by delaying sexual maturity and reducing the ultimate adult size achieved. Despite these important interrelationships it is difficult to recommend precisely what any one individual adolescent should eat.

It is even more difficult to obtain the adolescent's cooperation in any adult-determined regimen. An interested young person can be made aware of what the current recommendations are and what foods would meet those recommendations. As for the larger masses, most seem to muddle through reasonably well and somehow satisfy their nutritional needs in much the same erratic fashion they come to grips with the psychological changes necessary to move from the protected world of childhood to the independent world of the adult.

BIBLIOGRAPHY

Barnes, H. V. Physical growth and development during puberty. *Med Clin. N. Amer.* **59**:1305 (1975).

Cheek, D. B. Body composition, hormones, nutrition, and adolescent growth. In *The Control of the Onset of Puberty*. M. M. Grumbach, G. D. Grave, and F. E. Mayer, Eds., Wiley, New York, 1974.

Faiman, C., and Winter, J. S. D. Gonadotropins and sex hormone patterns in puberty, clinical data. In *The Control of the Onset of Puberty*. M. M. Grumbach, G. D. Grave, and F. E. Mayer, Eds., Wiley, New York, 1974.

Flynn, M. A., Clark, J., Reid, J. C., and Chase, G. A longitudinal study of total body potassium in normal children. *Pediat. Res.* **9**:834 (1975).

Forbes, G. B. Growth of lean body mass in man. *Growth* **36**:325 (1972).

Frisch, R. E. Critical weight at menarche, initiation of the adolescent growth spurt, and control of puberty. In *The Control of the Onset of Puberty*. M. M. Grumbach, G. D. Grave, and F. E. Mayer, Eds., Wiley, New York, 1974.

Heald, F. P. Adolescent nutrition. *Med. Clin. N. Amer.* **59**:1329 (1975).

Johnston, F. E., Roche, A. F., Schell, L. M., and Wettenhall, H. N. B. Critical weight at menarche. Critique of a hypothesis. *Am. J. Dis. Child.* **129**:19 (1975).

Marshall, W. A. Growth and sexual maturation in normal puberty. *Clin. Endocrin. Metab.* **4**:3 (1975).

Marshall, W. A., and Tanner, J. M. Variations in the pattern of pubertal changes in girls. *Arch. Dis. Child.* **44**:291 (1969).

Marshall, W. A., and Tanner, J. M. Variations in the pattern of pubertal changes in boys. *Arch. Dis. Child.* **45**:13 (1970).

National Research Council. Recommended Dietary Allowances, 8th ed. National Academy of Sciences, Washington, D.C., 1974.

Reiter, E. O., and Root, A. W. Hormonal changes of adolescence. *Med. Clin. N. Amer.* **59**:1289 (1975).

Tanner, J. M. *Growth at Adolescence*, 2nd ed. Blackwell, Oxford, 1962.

Tanner, J. M. Sequence and tempo in the somatic changes in puberty. In *The Control of the Onset of Puberty*. M. M. Grumbach, G. D. Grave, and F. E. Mayer, Eds., Wiley, New York, 1974.

Tanner, J. M. Growth and Endocrinology of the Adolescent. In *Endocrine and Genetic Diseases of Childhood*. Saunders, Philadelphia, 1969.

5

Nutrition and Lactation

ELSIE M. WIDDOWSON

Department of Investigative Medicine, University of Cambridge, England

In this chapter I shall discuss the cost of lactation to the organism, the special nutritional requirements caused by the physiological changes that occur during lactation, and the scientific data which demonstrate that proper nutrition is necessary for proper lactation. I shall also consider two other closely linked topics. The first concerns the changes that take place in the mother's body during pregnancy, which are partly required for the normal development of the fetus and partly in preparation for the subsequent demands of lactation. The second is the nutrition of the mother who produces a baby but does not breast-feed it, for that is the situation among many American mothers today.

THE COST OF LACTATION TO THE MOTHER

The mammary glands synthesize the milk from simple substances extracted from the plasma, glucose, amino acids, fatty acids, and minerals. The cost of lactation to the mother, therefore, includes not only the nutrients in the milk and their energy value, but also the energy required to synthesize the lactose, protein, and fat. It used to be thought that the energy efficiency of milk production was no more than 60% (1). Hytten and Thomson (2) produced evidence that the efficiency of milk production is nearer 80%, and the current NRC report (3) has accepted this figure. However Thomson, Hytten, and Billewicz (4) have published evidence of an even higher efficiency of 90%. Table 1 shows the daily volume of milk taken by infants of various ages and its energy value. The figures are based on the 50th percentile intakes given by

Table 1 Energy Cost of Producing Breast Milk

Age of Baby (months)	Volume of Milk Taken (ml/day)	Energy Value of Milk (kcal)	Total Energy Cost of Producing Milk Assuming 90% Efficiency (kcal/day)
0–1	600	402	446
1–2	840	563	626
2–3	930	623	692
3–4	960	643	714
4–5	1010	677	752
5–6	1100	737	819

Fomon (5), and assume that the infant is fully breast-fed. The third column of figures shows the total energy cost to the mother of producing these volumes of milk, assuming that the efficiency of milk production is 90%. These suggest that the lactating mother should have 600 to 800 kcal a day in addition to her normal daily intake. The current NRC report (3) recommends 500 kcal and the United Kingdom recommendation is also an extra 500 kcal (6). This is less than the energy cost of producing the milk, but it is assumed that some of the energy requirement will come from the mother's stores, which will be discussed below.

Table 2 gives representative amounts of protein, fat, carbohydrate, calcium, magnesium, phosphorus, iron, copper, zinc, vitamins A and C, thiamin, nicotinic acid, and riboflavin in 950 ml of breast milk which as we have seen is the mean volume taken by babies three months old. The NRC recommendations (3) for these nutrients for a nonlactating woman are given for comparison, with the supplement for lactation. The nutrients that make the greatest demand on the mother, in relation to her own intake, are calcium and vitamins A and C. The relation between the intake of vitamins by the mother and their concentration in the milk will be discussed later.

CHANGES IN THE MOTHER'S BODY DURING PREGNANCY AND LACTATION

An important physiological change in the mother's body during pregnancy is the deposition of fat. It has been estimated that a woman lays down about 4 kg of fat during a normal full-term pregnancy (7). This is a lot of fat. It weighs more than the average baby and may add over a third to the total

Table 2 Protein and Minerals in 950 ml Milk Compared with Recommended Allowances for a Woman, with the Supplement for Lactation

		Recommended Allowance	
	In 950 ml Milk	Woman	Lactation Supplement
Protein (g)	12	46	20
Calcium (mg)	330	800	400
Magnesium (mg)	40	300	150
Phosphorus (mg)	150	800	400
Iron (mg)	1.5	18	0
Zinc (mg)	5	15	10
Vitamin A (μg)	551	800	400
Vitamin C (mg)	41	45	35
Thiamin (mg)	0.15	1.1	0.3
Nicotinic acid (mg)	1.5	14	4
Riboflavin (mg)	0.4	1.4	0.5

amount of fat the mother had in her body before she became pregnant. Animals too deposit fat in their bodies during pregnancy. Rats were found to have 51 g of body fat before they were mated, and 72 g after delivery of their litters. Three weeks later, after suckling their litters, the female rats' bodies contained only 29 g (8). Women who breast-feed their babies probably lose most of their additional fat unless they maintain a very high intake of food, but this they find it difficult to do in the ordinary way, and the 36,000 kcal of energy stored by the woman during pregnancy in 4 kg of fat helps to provide for the energy requirements of the young. Even so, the mother must eat some extra food, and a small animal with a large weight of young like the rat must eat a great deal more food during lactation to provide for the synthesis of the milk required by the young. In fact, more food is eaten by rats during full lactation than after lesions have been made in the hypothalamus and they are rapidly becoming obese. There is considerable enlargement of the digestive tract, which has to deal with all the extra food, and the small intestine almost doubles in weight, though it does not increase in length (9). The liver also increases in size, and Fig. 1 shows the results of Kennedy, Pearce, and Parrott (10) for the weight of the livers of rats after delivery of their first litters, and after 10 and 21 days of lactation; it also shows the liver weights 14 and 21 days after the litters were weaned. The graph demonstrates the effect of the number of young in the litter, and therefore of the amount of milk produced and the amount of additional food eaten by the mother, on

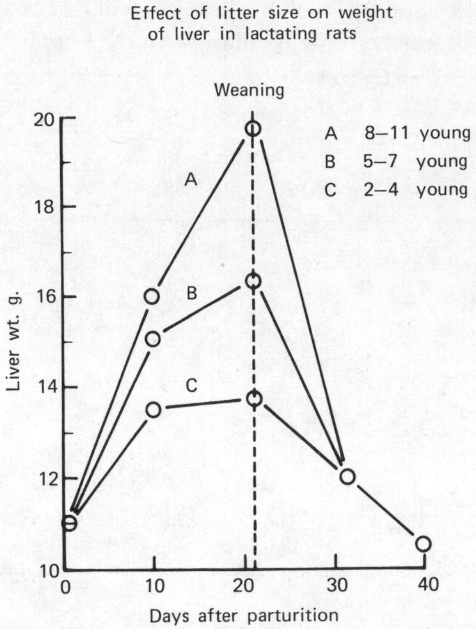

Figure 1. Effect of litter size on weight of liver in lactating rats.

growth of the liver. When there were 8 to 11 young in the litter the liver doubled in size.

Table 3 shows the protein and DNA content of the livers of these rats of Kennedy and co-workers (10). The amount of protein nearly doubled during lactation. The DNA increased, but not by so much, so that growth was due to an increase in both size and number of liver cells. After lactation was over, and the animals were eating less food, the size of the liver was reduced and so was the amount of protein in it, but there was no decrease in the amount of

Table 3 Effect of an Increased Food Intake Resulting from Lactation on the Amount of Protein and DNA in the Liver of Rats[a]

	Liver Weight (g)	Protein (mg)	DNA (mg)
Controls	6.9	1360	15.2
At end of first lactation	12.7	2340	19.4
Parous. Not lactating	7.7	1520	18.5

[a] From Kennedy *et al.* (10).

DNA or in the number of liver cells. Whether similar changes go on in the digestive tracts and livers of lactating women we do not know; if so, the magnitude of the growth will probably be considerably less.

Long and careful balance experiments on pregnant women made in the 1930s by Macy and her colleagues and by Coons and her co-workers suggested that considerably more nitrogen, calcium, phosphorus, and magnesium was retained by the mother than was required for the body of the fetus and for the enlargement of the tissues directly associated with the pregancy, i.e., the uterus, the placenta, and the mammary glands. The average total accumulation of nitrogen, for example, between the fourth and the tenth month of pregnancy was 515 g (11). Of this, 145 g were in tissues known to be concerned in the pregnancy, but 370 g of nitrogen or 2.3 kg of protein remained unaccounted for. It is difficult to see where so much protein, equivalent to 7 kg of lean tissue, could be stored. Hytten and Leitch (7) are probably correct in believing that these seemingly high retentions were due to cumulative errors inherent in the metabolic balance technique. These authors believe that no more protein is laid down in the mother's body than can be accounted for in the fetus, the uterus, the placenta, and the mammary glands. The same probably holds for the inorganic substances.

The amount of calcium contained in 950 ml of breast milk (330 mg) is considerable, but it would be provided by an extra pint and a quarter of cow's milk per day, provided that 50% of the calcium in the milk was absorbed. Women accustomed to living on low-calcium diets must absorb a considerably higher percentage than this, for Walker and co-workers (12) found no X-ray evidence of skeletal demineralization in Bantu women with seven or more children, compared with similar women with two or fewer children. The average intake of calcium by both groups was only 300 to 400 mg per day. The explanation has become clear as a result of the recent work on the active metabolite of vitamin D, 1, 25-dihydrocholecalciferol, which is secreted by the kidney (13). It initiates the synthesis of a specific calcium-binding protein in the cytoplasm of the small intestine, which serves for the active transport of calcium across the gut (14). This transport is regulated by calcitonin and parathyroid hormone, and in times of greater calcium need, as in lactating women with low calcium intakes, a high proportion of dietary calcium will be transported across the intestine.

THE NUTRITION OF THE MOTHER WHO DOES NOT BREAST-FEED HER BABY

The mother who does not breast-feed her baby has an extra 4 kg or so of fat inside her after her baby is born and the question is, what happens to this fat?

Naismith and Ritchie (15) have tried to find out. They followed the body weights, skinfold thicknesses and energy intakes of 22 women who fully breast-fed their babies to three months, and of 20 women who did not breast-feed at all. Both groups lost about 3 kg of weight during the three months; those not lactating achieved the loss by eating considerably less food than those that were breast-feeding, the energy intakes being 2000 and 2900 kcal per day, respectively. Mothers who did not lactate consciously restricted their food intakes. There is no doubt that a restricted food intake or increased activity or both is the only way to get rid of the additional fat. One other interesting point emerged from this study. There was very little change in skinfold measurements, and this suggests that the fat laid down during pregnancy is deposited around the internal organs and not underneath the skin.

THE EFFECT OF ALTERATIONS IN THE AMOUNTS OF WATER, ENERGY, AND NUTRIENTS IN THE MOTHER'S DIET ON THE VOLUME AND COMPOSITION OF HER MILK

The effect of the mother's intake of water on milk secretion is in the opposite direction from what one might expect. Illingworth and Kilpatrick (16) showed that drinking water in amounts larger than those the mother wishes to drink to quench her thirst actually impairs lactation. This impairment is thought to be due to the suppression of posterior pituitary secretion. On the other hand dehydration reduces milk secretion only when the volume drunk is less than the volume of milk secreted.

A low intake of energy during pregnancy or lactation reduces the volume of milk secreted, but it does not of itself affect the composition. There are many accounts in the literature of the inability of women to breast-feed their babies in times of famine, for example, during the siege of Paris (17) and the siege of Lenigrad (18). Dean (19) was able to make a quantitative study of this in Germany after World War II. He analyzed the records of 22,000 births at the Landesfrauen Klinik, Wuppertal, during the years 1937 to 1948. In 1937 and 1938, before the war started, there was food in plenty, but in 1945 to 1946 food was in very short supply. The average volume of milk produced on the seventh day was 390 ml in 1937 compared with 290 ml in 1945. Studies on animals, for example pigs and rats, have always led to the same conclusion (20, 21). When female rats that have been severely undernourished are rehabilitated, their lactation performance is completely restored (21), and we have found the same to be true of pigs. The pigs were so severely undernourished that at one year they weighed only 5 kg instead of the normal 150 mg. If they were then rehabilitated the females produced normal young and provided sufficient milk for them to grow at a perfectly normal rate. The evidence shows that the same is true for women. In contrast to this there is no evidence that obese women produce more milk than women of more normal dimensions.

There is wide individual variation among women in the volume and composition of the milk they produce. Table 4 shows the ranges for the concentration of some of the constituents of milk as given by Macy and Kelly (22).

Table 4 Variation in Composition of Mature Milk Between Individual Women[a] (per 100 ml)

	Minimum	Maximum
Energy (kcal)	45	119
Protein (g)	0.7	2.0
Fat (g)	1.3	8.3
Carbohydrate (g)	5.0	9.2
Calcium (mg)	17	61
Phosphorus (mg)	7	27
Magnesium (mg)	2	6
Sodium (mg)	6	44
Potassium (mg)	37	64
Chloride (mg)	9	73

[a] From Macy & Kelly (22).

The samples were taken under controlled conditions of collection and analysis from women at the same stage of lactation living in the same geographical area and known to have been having an adequate diet. The range, particularly for some of the inorganic constituents, is very wide indeed.

Differences in the relative amounts of protein, fat, and carbohydrate in the mother's diet may influence the volume of milk secreted, but they do not affect the concentration of these nutrients in the milk (23). There have been reports of very low concentrations of protein in the milk of women in Bangalore (24), Papua (25), and Pakistan (26). It is impossible from the evidence to determine whether these low concentrations are attributable to climate or racial differences, to diet, or to some other cause.

The amounts of the inorganic constituents in the mother's diet do not correlate well with the concentrations in the milk. On the other hand the amounts of the various vitamins in the woman's diet greatly influence the concentrations of them in her milk. For example, Tarjan and co-workers (27) showed that eating liver at one meal was sufficient to double the concentration of vitamin A in the milk within eight hours. Additional vitamin C, thiamin, and riboflavin taken by the mother all cause a temporary rise in the concentration of the vitamin in the milk (28, 29).

Thus all evidence shows that breast milk is not a secretion of constant composition. It varies from woman to woman, possibly with race or climate, and certainly with stage of lactation and some constituents of the mother's diet. Nevertheless, it remains the best food for the baby.

REFERENCES

1. National Research Council Food and Nutrition Board. Recommended Dietary Allowances, 7th ed. National Academy of Sciences, Washington, D.C., 1968.
2. Hytten, F. E. and Thomson, A. M. In *Milk: The Mammary Gland and its Secretion*. Vol. 2. S. K. Kon and A. T. Cowie, Eds., Academic, New York, 1961, p. 3.
3. National Research Council Food and Nutrition Board. Recommended Dietary Allowances 8th Revised ed. National Academy of Sciences, Washington, D.C., 1974.
4. Thomson, A. M., Hytten, F. E., and Billewicz, W. Z. *Br. J. Nutr.* **24**:565 (1970).
5. Fomon, S. J. *Infant Nutrition*, 2nd ed. Saunders, Philadelphia, 1974.
6. Department of Health and Social Security. Reports on Public Health and Medical Subjects No. 120. HMSO, London (1969).
7. Hytten, F. E. and Leitch, I. *The Physiology of Human Pregnancy*, 2nd ed. Blackwell, Oxford, 1971.
8. Spray, C. M. *Br. J. Nutr.* **4**:354 (1950).
9. Barnett, S. A. and Widdowson, E. M. *J. Reprod. Fert.* **26**:39 (1971).
10. Kennedy, G. C., Pearce, W. M., and Parrott, D. M. V. *J. Endoc.*, **17**:158 (1958).
11. Macy, I. G. and Hunscher, H. A. *Am. J. Obstet.* **27**:878 (1934).
12. Walker, A. R. P., Richardson, B., and Walker, F. *Clin. Sci.*, **42**:189 (1972).
13. Lawson, D. E. M., Fraser, D. R., Kodicek, E., Morris, H. R., and Williams, D. H. *Nature*, Lond., **230**:228 (1971).
14. De Luca, H. F. *Proc. Fed. Am. Soc. Exp. Biol.*, **28**:1678 (1969).
15. Naismith, D. J. and Ritchie, C. D. *Proc. Nutr. Soc.*, **34**:116A (1975).
16. Illingworth, R. S. and Kilpatrick, B. *Lancet*, **265**:1175 (1953).
17. Descaine, M. E. *Gaz. méd. Fr.*, **26**:317 (1871).
18. Antonov, A. N. *J. Pediat.* **30**:250 (1947).
19. Dean, R. F. A. Spec. Rep. Ser. Med. Coun. No. 275, p. 346 HMSO, London (1951).
20. Rook, J. A. F. and Witter, R. *Proc. Nutr. Soc.*, **27**:71 (1968).
21. Widdowson, E. M. and Cowen, J. *Br. J. Nutr.* **27**:85 (1972).
22. Macy, I. G. and Kelly, H. J. In *Milk: The Mammary Gland and its Secretion*, Vol. 2. S. K. Kon and A. T. Cowie, Eds., Academic, New York, 1961, p. 265.
23. Gunther, M. and Stanier, J. Spec. Rep. Ser. Med. Res. Coun. No. 275, HMSO, London (1951).

24. Deb, A. K. and Cama, H. R. *Br. J. Nutr.*, **16**:65 (1962).

25. Jansen, A. A. J., Luyken, R., Malcolm, S. H., and Willems, J. J. L. *Trop. Geog. Med.*, **12**:138 (1960).

26. Lindblad, B. S. and Rahimtoola, R. *Acta Paediat. Stock.*, **63**:125 (1974).

27. Tarjan, R., Kramer, M., Szöke, K., and Lindner, K. *Nutritio Dieta*, **5**:12 (1963).

28. Kon, S. K. and Mawson, E. M. Spec. Rep. Ser. Med. Res. Coun. No. 269 HMSO, London (1950).

29. Deodhar, A. D., Rajalakshmi, R., and Ramakrishnan, C. V. *Acta Paediat. Stock.*, **53**:42 (1964).

PART 3

Special Nutrition Problems

6

Anemias

VICTOR HERBERT, M.D., J.D.

Departments of Pathology and Medicine, Columbia University College of Physicians and Surgeons; Hematology and Nutrition Laboratory, Veterans Administration Hospital, Bronx, New York

Anemia is defined as a reduction below normal in the amount of red blood which occurs when the equilibrium between blood production and blood loss (through bleeding or destruction) is disturbed (1). By World Health Organization criteria (2), anemia is considered to exist when the nonpregnant female has a hemoglobin below 12 and the pregnant adult female a hemoglobin below 11 g per 100 ml of venous blood (when at sea level; normal values are higher at higher altitudes). The observations of Scott, Pritchard, and associates (3) indicate that the hemoglobin concentration of healthy nonpregnant young women without iron deficiency will almost always be 12 g/100 ml or more, that at midpregnancy this value will practically always be at least 10 g/100 ml, but fairly often may be less than 11 g/100 ml, and that late in pregnancy this figure will almost always be 10 g/100 ml or more, in the absence of iron deficiency. The normal fall of hemoglobin during pregnancy is simply pregnancy hypervolemia (which increases both the plasma and the red cell volume, with a greater increase in the former).

Nutritional anemia is defined as a condition in which the hemoglobin content of the blood is lower than normal as a result of a deficiency of one or more essential nutrients. To delineate a given anemia as nutritional, two criteria must be met: lack of the nutrient must produce, and providing the

Supported in part by United States Public Health Service Grant AM15163, and in part by a Veterans Administration Medical Investigatorship (3570–01 and 3570–02) to Dr. Herbert.

nutrient must correct, the anemia. By these two criteria there are only three unequivocal nutritional anemias: those due to lack of iron, lack of folate, or lack of vitamin B_{12} (4). These three anemias reflect an important nutritional problem affecting large population groups, particularly the poverty-stricken and those under metabolic stress.

Iron deficiency and folate deficiency are more common in women because of two forms of metabolic stress peculiar to women: the monthly blood loss in premenopausal women and the drain on maternal nutrient stores imposed by pregnancy. The fetus will take from the mother whatever it needs in order to be born normal, even if this produces severe nutrient deficiency in the mother (5). Since anemia is a relatively late manifestation of nutritional deficiency, those patients diagnosed as having nutritional anemia are the "tip of the iceberg"—part of a larger group suffering from nutrient depletion of more moderate degree which is not yet manifest by unequivocal anemia.

The metabolic stress of menstrual blood loss is increased by the use of some intrauterine contraceptive devices (6, 7) and decreased by the use of oral contraceptives (8). In fact, advertising of "unique vitamin-mineral formulas for the special needs of patients taking oral contraceptives" is misleading because it has not been established that there is any such special need (8, 9).

IRON DEFICIENCY ANEMIA

About one-third to one-half of apparently healthy young American women have laboratory evidence of iron depletion (10–12). Sturgeon and Shoden (12) found less than 5 mg of iron per 100 g of liver tissue in 40% of women age 20 to 50, indicative of iron depletion. This was true of only 13% of women over age 50 (and less than 10% of all men). It should be noted that iron depletion (loss of body iron stores) precedes anemia. While a majority of women who are anemic have iron deficiency, this is not always the case, so blanket treatment of every anemic woman with iron, without ascertaining that she in fact has iron deficiency, can do positive harm (for example, in women with sickle cell or other hemolytic anemias with increased iron stores, in whom the giving of iron may produce "iron overload" syndrome). Nevertheless, the incidence of anemia in various groups of American pregnant women has ranged from 10 to 60%, most of which could be prevented by prophylactic iron therapy (13).

Menstrual loss of iron is the main source of the iron losses in nonpregnant women in the fertile age group (14, 15). The average menstrual blood loss is about 40 ml/cycle (15), representing a loss of about 20 mg of iron per cycle. About 10% of women have menorrhagia, with a blood loss exceeding 80 ml/

cycle (16), making them particularly susceptible to iron deficiency. The use of more than 12 pads during a menstrual period, or the damming up of blood behind tampons, suggests excessive menstrual bleeding (15, 17).

The situation of American women with respect to iron balance is more clearly understood from Tables 1 and 2, which present, respectively, the estimated dietary iron requirements of Americans (Table 1) and the iron requirements of pregnant American women (Table 2). The absorbability of iron from different food sources is highly variable, with an average absorption of

Table 1 Estimated Dietary Iron Requirements[a]

	Absorbed Iron Requirement (mg/day)	Dietary Iron Requirement[b] (mg/day)
Normal men and nonmenstruating women	0.5–1	5–10
Menstruating women	0.7–2	7–20
Pregnant women	2–4.8	20–48[c]
Adolescents	1–2	10–20
Children	0.4–1	4–10
Infants	0.5–1.5	1.5 mg/kg[d]

[a] After (13). Courtesy of the *Journal of the American Medical Association.*
[b] Assuming 10% absorption.
[c] This amount of iron cannot be derived from diet and should be met by iron supplementation in the latter half of pregnancy.
[d] To a maximum of 15 mg.

Table 2 Iron Requirements for Pregnancy[a]

	Average (mg)	Range (mg)
External iron loss	170	150–200
Expansion of red blood cell mass	450	200–600
Fetal iron	270	200–370
Iron in placenta and cord	90	30–170
Blood loss at delivery	150	90–310
Total requirement[b]	980	580–1340
Cost of pregnancy[c]	680	440–1050

[a] After (13). Courtesy of the *Journal of the American Medical Association.*
[b] Blood loss at delivery not included.
[c] Expansion of red cell mass not included.

about 10% of the total iron in the diet (18). Therefore, the amount of iron ingested must be ten times the daily requirement, as Table 1 indicates. Since the average American diet provides about 6 mg of iron per thousand kcal (10), iron intake from dietary sources is borderline for teenage girls and women, and may be inadequate for infants and pregnant women (13, 19). Nevertheless, a woman who has sufficient iron stores to provide for her increase in hemoglobin mass during pregnancy, and who breast-feeds her infant for six months (thereby delaying the return of menstruation), will have her iron needs covered by an adequate intake of dietary iron (20).

The diagnostic features of iron deficiency are summarized in Table 3 (21). To this table should be added the fact that 5 mg or less of iron per 100 g of liver tissue indicates depletion of the storage pool to the extent that iron deficiency anemia may be either present or anticipated with any further depletion (12).

Table 3 Sequential Changes (from Left to Right) in the Development of Iron Deficiency[a]

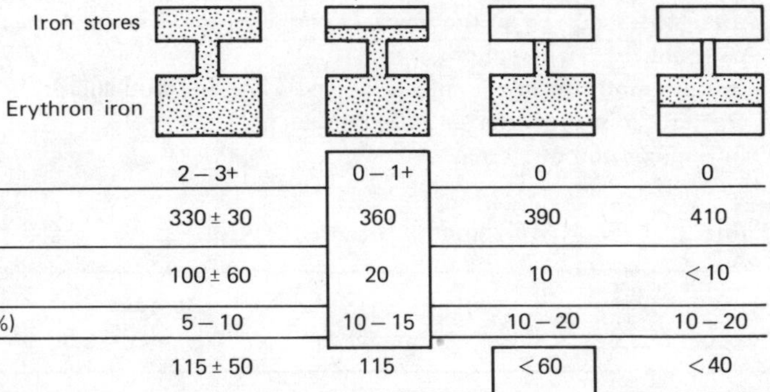

	Normal	Iron depletion	Iron–deficient erythropoiesis	Iron–deficiency anemio
RE marrow Fe	2 – 3+	0 – 1+	0	0
Transferrin IBC (μg/100 ml)	330 ± 30	360	390	410
Plasma ferritin (ng/ml)	100 ± 60	20	10	< 10
Iron absorption (%)	5 – 10	10 – 15	10 – 20	10 – 20
Plasma iron (μg/100 ml)	115 ± 50	115	< 60	< 40
Transferrin saturation (%)	35 ± 15	30	< 15	< 10
Sideroblasts (%)	40 – 60	40–60	< 10	< 10
RBC protoporphyrin (μg/100 ml RBC)	30	30	100	200
Erythrocytes	Normal	Normal	Normal	Microcytic/ hypochromic

[a] Rectangles enclose the first appearance of the indicated abnormal test results. IBC is the iron-binding capacity. After (21) courtesy of F. A. Davis Co.

As stated in the footnote to Table 1, the amount of iron required to meet the needs of pregnancy should usually be met by iron supplementation in the second half of pregnancy, since it cannot usually be derived from the diet. The Committee on Maternal Nutrition (5) recommends supplementation with 30 to 60 mg of iron daily (i.e., 150 to 300 mg of ferrous sulfate) during pregnancy. The physician should use his judgment in this regard, based on knowledge of the patient, the dietary habits, the fact that iron deficiency is frequent in pregnant women, and the blood and iron status of the particular patient (22, 23). He may routinely give iron (24).

In general, oral ferrous sulfate, the least expensive iron preparation, is the drug of choice for treating iron deficiency. A detailed discussion of iron therapy is presented elsewhere (22, 23). It is important to remember that the duration of oral therapy for iron deficiency should be approximately six months, since therapy for a shorter time will not adequately replete body iron stores. The physician must remember that the iron deficiency may have developed in association with menorrhagia. If that menorrhagia persists, iron therapy may have to persists as well so that the iron loss in blood does not again produce a negative iron balance.

FOLATE DEFICIENCY ANEMIA

Studies carried out under the aegis of the World Health Organization (2, 20) in various countries suggest that up to one-third of all the pregnant women in the world have folate deficiency. In a recent study in a New York City municipal clinic, our group (25) found tissue deficiency of folic acid, as measured by a red cell folate level below 150 ng/ml, in 16% of 110 sequential pregnant women at the time of their first prenatal visit to the clinic. An additional 14% had red cell folate levels in the range "suggestive but not conclusive for tissue folate depletion" (150 to 199 ng/ml).

These studies add to a growing body of evidence that nutritional deficiency of folic acid is prevalent among Americans of poor economic status. Based on findings up to 1970, Pritchard, writing for the Committee on Maternal Nutrition of the Food and Nutrition Board (5), recommended that folic acid supplements should be taken throughout pregnancy. Subsequently, the data of the Ten-State Nutrition Survey of 1968–1970 became available (26). Although that survey found that "the mean serum folate values were, with few exceptions, above the acceptable level of 6 ng/ml and the mean red cell folate values were in the acceptable range of 150 to 650 ng/ml," a more detailed evaluation indicates that a real problem in fact exists, obscured by the use of mean values alone (25). The mean values obscured the existence of a substantial number of actual values sufficiently below the mean as to suggest widespread folic acid deficiency. This is indicated by the data from the Survey Director for Massachusetts of the Ten-State Nutrition Survey (27).

In Massachusetts, serum and red cell folates were measured on most of the samples collected. Of all the 1087 Massachusetts blood samples from females on which such measurements were made, 25.6% had red cell folate values below 150 ng/ml. This includes 115 pregnant women in the economically poor Roxbury-Dorchester area, all of whom were receiving prenatal clinic care, and most of whom were receiving vitamin supplements, presumably containing folic acid. Among these pregnant women, 7.1% had red cell folate values below 160 ng/ml and 7.1% had serum folate levels below 3 ng/ml. It is probably relevant that the more than 10,000 individuals surveyed in Massachusetts were randomly selected from enumeration districts with the lowest average income (lowest quartile) according to the 1960 census (26) and poverty and folate deficiency tend to run hand in hand (28, 29). As the Massachusetts report noted (27), "The results suggest that the diets currently eaten by a large segment of the population cannot provide the allowance of folic acid recommended for optimal health and, therefore, that dietary deficiency of folic acid may pose a major nutritional problem. If these findings are considered together with the finding of a high prevalence of low plasma vitamin A levels, it would appear that these diets contain insufficient amounts of green leafy vegetables which are major sources of both folic acid and provitamin A. Current processes for preservation, storage, and preparation of foods may also destroy a high proportion of the folate in foods."

The hazard to mother and fetus of folate deficiency in the absence of frank anemia is unclear and has been extensively reviewed (30). Studies from South Africa suggest that folate supplements in this situation decrease the incidence of prematurity (31) and cause significant elevation of hemoglobin levels (32–34), suggesting that even mild deficiency may limit DNA synthesis. Prospective studies of the effects on the fetus are difficult to interpret because folate administration invariably starts only after the period of maximum fetal susceptibility in the first trimester. However, animal experiments demonstrate a consistent teratogenic effect of folate deprivation from the time of conception, dependent on the duration of the experiment (25).

Hence, in the light of present knowledge it appears appropriate to correct folate deficiency in pregnancy. The implementation of this principle by improving the quality and quantity of available food is a long-term ideal limited by custom and economic circumstances. For this reason, the Joint FAO/WHO Expert Committee on Nutrition has recommended that food fortification should be considered as an immediate possibility for the improvement of intake of any deficient nutrient (35). A series of studies indicate that fortification of staple foods with folic acid is feasible, safe, effective, and in accordance with the recommendations of the Expert Committee (32–34, 36–

38). With adequate fortification, the possible hazards of folate deficiency in early pregnancy would be averted. Until such fortification is practiced, administration of folic acid tablets, 200 to 400 μg/day, is appropriate for all pregnant women, with 300 μg probably adequate for any pregnant population group (39).

The evidence relating folate deficiency in pregnancy to mental retardation and other defects in central nervous system function and development in the offspring is reviewed elsewhere (40). Currently available evidence is far from conclusive, but does constitute one more slight increment in the balance favoring the concept of daily folate supplementation throughout pregnancy.

A National Academy of Sciences "Workshop on Human Folate Requirements," whose proceedings are currently being prepared for publication, included papers presenting the latest information on distribution of folates in food, food folate availability, results of several surveys to detect folate deficiency in certain American population groups, and reviews of the folic acid requirement in children, in adults, and in situations of increased need. To summarize the findings most pertinent to nutritional anemias in American women, measurement of serum and red cell folate together constitutes the best method for delineating the existence of folate deficiency; food folate availability is affected by various constituents present in different foodstuffs; pregnancy increases the folate requirement.

The minimal daily adult requirement for folic acid which must be absorbed from food to sustain normality is in the range of 50 μg daily (28),

Table 4 Effect of Oral Contraceptive Agents (OCA) on Folacin and B_{12} Levels in Blood[a]

	Group	N	Mean	±SD	% Deficient	% Low
Serum folacin (> 5.0 ng/ml[b]; < 3.0 ng/ml[c])	OCA	80	4.5	2.0	17	54
	Non-OCA	71	5.4[d]	2.4	14	34
Red cell folacin (140–650 ng/ml packed cells[b])	OCA	70	172.8	56.9		30
	Non-OCA	64	199.4[d]	62.3		9
Serum vitamin B_{12} (> 0.2 ng/ml[b])	OCA	77	0.48	0.24		7
	Non-OCA	72	0.69[e]	0.29		2

[a] From (41).
[b] Acceptable level.
[c] Deficient level.
[d] $p < .02$.
[e] $p < .01$.

and the Food and Nutrition Board (19) recommends that the diet of adults contain 400 μg daily. This requirement appears to be approximately doubled by pregnancy. Thus, if a woman is absorbing from her food in the range of 100 μg of folic acid daily from the start of pregnancy, she may not need supplementation, but assuming lesser stores than normal at the start of pregnancy, and supplementation beginning later than the start of pregnancy, 200 to 300 μg of folate supplementation daily may be necessary (22, 23, 39). The Food and Nutrition Board (19) recommends a daily dietary intake of 800 μg during pregnancy and 600 μg during lactation.

Table 5 Levels of Plasma and Erythrocyte Folic Acid in OCA Users[a]

Economic Level and Hormone Use	Plasma Folic Acid (ng/ml)			Erythrocyte Folic Acid (ng/ml)		
	S	NS	Avg.	S	NS	Avg.
A-none	6.74 ±4.70	5.55 ±3.09	6.20 ±4.19	322 ±180	270 ±109	303 ±159
A-1	3.38 ±0.82	3.97 ±1.61	3.81 ±1.44	201 ±74	170 ±40	178 ±50
A-2	4.60 ±0.76	4.76 ±3.30	4.72 ±2.86	245 ±115	189 ±106	200 ±109
A-RP	1.57 ±15.99	3.35 ±0.65	9.87 ±12.31	700 ±420	177 ±58	401 ±372
B-None	3.72 ±0.99	3.49 ±1.12	4.14 ±2.51	238 ±94	171 ±70	185 ±78
B-1	4.15 ±3.49	4.13 ±1.65	4.14 ±2.07	241 ±186	206 ±99	213 ±120
B-2	5.00 ±1.38	3.70 ±1.20	3.97 ±1.38	204 ±89	174 ±73	139 ±76
B-RP	6.24 ±7.30	4.23 ±1.75	4.77 ±4.08	274 ±265	244 ±166	252 ±197
p values		S .001 I .001			p_2 .001 Ip_1 .06 Ip_2 .04 I .01 S .001	

[a] From (42). Values are mean ± standard deviation of mean. S = Supplemented; NS = Nonsupplemented; Avg = Average. A is higher and B is lower economic status. None = no oral contraceptive. 1 and 2 = two different oral contraceptives. RP = resumed oral contraceptives after pregnancy.

Although serum and red cell folate may be lowered by the use of oral contraceptives (41, 42) (see Tables 4 and 5), it is not yet clear that folate supplementation is needed by women taking such products (8, 43). This folate need would probably be adequately met by one fresh uncooked vegetable, fruit, or fruit juice daily (22, 23).

VITAMIN B_{12}

Although the serum vitamin B_{12} level falls in pregnancy (44) and may also fall with the use of oral contraceptives (41, 45), tissue levels of vitamin B_{12} may remain normal and vitamin B_{12} deficiency anemia has not seemed to be a problem (45). From evidence so far, American women do not seem substantially more likely than men to have vitamin B_{12} deficiency anemia (22, 23). Nevertheless, in population groups where vitamin B_{12} deficiency is common due to vegetarianism, such vitamin B_{12} deficiency would be increased by the metabolic stress of pregnancy, including the fetal drain on maternal stores of about 0.3 μg of B_{12} per day (20, 28), and by a mean of 0.3 μg of B_{12} per day lost in breast milk during lactation (20). It is for these reasons that the Recommended Dietary Allowance (19) for vitamin B_{12} was raised from the 3 μg for adults in general to 4 μg for pregnant or lactating adults.

REFERENCES

1. *Dorland's Illustrated Medical Dictionary* (25th Ed.). Saunders, Philadelphia, 1974.
2. WHO Scientific Group. *Nutritional Anaemias.* WHO Tech. Rept. Ser. No. 405, 1968. Purchasable for $1.00 from Publication Distribution and Sales, World Health Organization, 1211 Geneva 27, Switzerland.
3. Scott, D. E., Pritchard, J. A., Saltin, A. S., and Humphreys, J. M. Iron deficiency during pregnancy. In *Iron Deficiency.* L. Hallberg, H.-G. Harwerth, and A. Vannotti, Eds. Academic, London and New York, 1970, pp. 491–503.
4. Herbert, V. Introduction to the nutritional anemias. *Seminars Hemat.* 7:2 (1970).
5. Committee on Maternal Nutrition. *Maternal Nutrition and the Course of Pregnancy.* Food and Nutrition Board, National Research Council, National Academy of Science, Washington, D.C., 1970.
6. Anonymous. Topical and systematic contraceptive agents. *Medical Letter* **16**:37 (1974).
7. Anonymous. Cu-7, a copper-containing IUD. *Medical Letter* **17**:26 (1975).
8. Anonymous. Feminins and other vitamin-mineral supplements for women taking oral contraceptives. *Medical Letter* **15**:81 (1973).
9. Symposium. Effects of oral contraceptive hormones on nutrient metabolism. *Am. J. Clin. Nutr.* **28**:333–402; 521–560 (1975).

10. Monsen, E. R., Kuhn, I. N., and Finch, C. A. Iron status of menstruating women. *Am. J. Clin. Nutr.* **20**:842 (1967).

11. Scott, D. E. and Pritchard, J. A. Iron deficiency in healthy young college women. *J.A.M.A.* **199**:897 (1967).

12. Sturgeon, P. and Shoden, A. Total liver storage iron in normal populations of the USA. *Am. J. Clin. Nutr.* **24**:469 (1971).

13. AMA Council on Foods and Nutrition. Iron deficiency in the United States. *J.A.M.A.* **203**:407 (1968).

14. Rybo, G. Menstrual loss of iron. In *Iron Deficiency*. L. Hallberg, H.-G. Howerth, and A. Vannotti, Eds. Academic, London and New York, 1970, pp. 163–171.

15. Fairbanks, V. F., Fahey, J. L., and Beutler, E., Eds. *Clinical Disorders of Iron Metabolism* (2nd Ed.) Grune and Stratton, New York and London, 1971.

16. Hallberg, L., Hogdahl, A.-M., Nilsson, L., and Rybo, G. Menstrual blood loss, a population study: Variation at different ages and attempts to define normality, 1966.

17. Moore, C. V. and Dubach, R. Metabolism and requirements of iron in the human. *J.A.M.A.* **162**:197 (1956).

18. Layrisse, M. Iron nutriture. In *Proceedings, Western Hemisphere Nutrition Congress IV*. P. L. White, and N. Selvey, Eds., Publishing Sciences Group, Acton, Mass., 1975, pp. 148–154.

19. Committee on Dietary Allowances. Recommended Dietary Allowances. Food and Nutrition Board, National Research Council, National Academy of Sciences. Washington, D.C., 1974.

20. F.A.O. and W.H.O. Expert Group. Requirements of Ascorbic Acid, Vitamin D, Vitamin B_{12}, Folate, and Iron. WHO Tech. Rept. Ser. No. 452, 1970. Purchasable for $1.25 from WHO in Geneva or American Public Health Assoc., 1740 Broadway, New York, N.Y. 11109. Available in English, French, Spanish, Russian, and Chinese.

21. Hillman, R. S. and Finch, C. A. *Red Cell Manual*. Davis, Philadelphia, 1974.

22. Herbert, V. Drugs effective in iron-deficiency and other hypochromic anemias. In *The Pharmacological Basis of Therapeutics*, 5th Ed. L. S. Goodman, and A. Gilman, Eds., Macmillan, New York. 1975, pp. 1324–1349.

24. Wallerstein, R. O. Iron metabolism and iron deficiency during pregnancy. *Clinics in Haemat.* **2**:453 (1973).

25. Herbert, V., Colman, N., Spivack, M., Ocasio, E., Ghanta, V., Kimmel, K., Brenner, L., Freundlich, J., and Scott, J. Folic acid deficiency in the United States: Folate assays in a prenatal clinic. *Am. J. Obstet. Gynecol.* **123**:175 (1975).

26. Ten-State Nutrition Survey 1968–70: U.S. Department of Health, Education and Welfare, Center for Disease Control. Atlanta, Ga. DHEW Publications No. (HSM) 72–8130 through 8134.

27. Edozien, J. C. National Nutrition Survey, Massachusetts, July 1969–June 1971, Report of the Survey Director to the Commissioner for Public Health, Commonwealth of Massachusetts, Boston, Mass., 1972. (Kindly supplied to us by Derek Robinson, M.D., Director, Division of Community Operations, Department of Public Health, Commonwealth of Mass.)

28. Herbert, V. Nutritional requirements of vitamin B_{12} and folic acid. *Am. J. Clin. Nutr.* **21**:743 (1968).

29. Kahn, S. B., Fein, S., Rigberg, S., and Brodsky, I. Correlation of folate metabolism and socioeconomic status in pregnancy and in patients taking oral contraceptives. *Am. J. Obstet. Gynecol.* **108**:931 (1970).

30. Rothman, D. Folic acid in pregnancy. *Am. J. Obstet. Gynecol.* **108**:149 (1970).

31. Baumslag, N., Edelstein, T., and Metz, J. Reduction of incidence of prematurity by folic acid supplementation in pregnancy. *Brit. Med. J.* **1**:16 (1970).

32. Colman, N., Green, R., and Metz, J. Prevention of folate deficiency by food fortification. II. Absorption of folic acid from fortified staple foods. *Am. J. Clin. Nutr.* **28**:459 (1975).

33. Colman, N., Barker, E. A., Barker, M., Green, R., and Metz, J. Prevention of folate deficiency by food fortification. IV. Identification of target groups in addition to pregnant women in an adult rural population. *Am. J. Clin. Nutr.* **28**:471 (1975).

34. Colman, N., Larsen, J. V., Barker, E. A., Green, R., and Metz, J. Prevention of folate deficiency by food fortification. III. Effect in pregnant subjects of varying amounts of added folic acid. *Am. J. Clin. Nutr.* **28**:465 (1975).

35. F.A.O. and W.H.O. Expert Committee on Nutrition. Food Fortification. World Health Organ. Tech. Rept. Ser. No. 477, 1971.

36. Colman, N., Barker, M., Green, R., and Metz, J. Prevention of folate deficiency in pregnancy by food fortification. *Am. J. Clin. Nutr.* **27**:339 (1974).

37. Colman, N., Green, R., Stevens, K., and Metz, J. Prevention of folate deficiency by food fortification. VI. The antimegaloblastic effect of folic acid-fortified maize meal. *S. African Med. J.* **48**:1795 (1974).

38. Colman, N., Larsen, J. V., Barker, M., Barker, E. A., Green, R., and Metz, J. Prevention of folate deficiency by food fortification. V. A pilot field trial of folic acid-fortified maize meal. *S. African Med. J.* **48**:1763 (1974).

39. Herbert, V. Folic acid requirement in adults. In *Workshop on Human Folate Requirements*. National Academy of Sciences, in press.

40. Herbert, V. and Tisman, G. Effects of deficiencies of folic acid and vitamin B_{12} on central nervous system function and development. In *Biology of Brain Dysfunction*, Vol. 1. G. Gaull, Ed., Plenum, New York and London, 1973, pp. 373–392.

41. Smith, J. L., Goldsmith, G. A., and Lawrence, J. D. Effects of oral contraceptive steroids on vitamin and lipid levels in serum. *Am. J. Clin. Nutr.* **28**:377 (1975).

42. Prasad, A. S., Lei, K. Y., Oberleas, D., Moghissi, K. S., and Stryker, J. C. Effect of oral contraceptive agents on nutrients. II. Vitamins. *Am. J. Clin. Nutr.* **28**:385 (1975).

43. Lindenbaum, J., Whitehead, N., and Reyner, F. Oral contraceptive hormones, folate metabolism, and the cervical epithelium. *Am. J. Clin. Nutr.* **28**:346 (1975).

44. Cooper, B. Folate and vitamin B_{12} in pregnancy. *Clinics in Haemat.* **2**:461 (1973).

45. Wertalik, L. F., Metz, E. N., LoBuglio, A. F., and Balcerzak, S. P. Decreased serum B_{12} levels with oral contraceptive use. *J.A.M.A.* **221**:1371 (1972).

7

Vitamins

R. B. ALFIN-SLATER

School of Public Health, University of California at Los Angeles

From the earliest days of recorded history man has been endowing certain nutrients in foods, especially vitamins, with properties and qualities above and beyond those which have been established as a result of extensive experimentation.

Vitamins, of course, are essential nutrients for man, woman, and many other species of animals. For the most part, they are incapable of being synthesized and need to be supplied in the diet. The amounts of vitamins A, D, and E and vitamins B_1, B_2, B_6, B_{12}, niacin, folic acid, and vitamin C required for good health in most of the population in the United States have been quantitatively identified and these values are given in a publication known as the Recommended Dietary Allowances (RDA). The RDA is the work of the Committee on Dietary Allowances of the Food and Nutrition Board, National Academy of Sciences, National Research Council. The latest edition appeared in 1974.

The recommendations for vitamins in many cases are different for men and for women. In some instances the difference is based on the fact that the requirement for vitamins is associated with caloric intake and because of their smaller stature and, in most cases, their lower amount of physical activity, women require fewer calories for the maintenance of good health. As a result, the RDA for vitamins A, E, niacin, riboflavin, and thiamin is lower for women than for men. However, for pregnant and lactating women, there is an increased requirement for vitamins A, E, C, B_6, B_{12}, folic acid, niacin, riboflavin, and thiamin. Similarly for women taking oral contraceptives a recent report on nutritional status and oral contraceptives (1) indicates that, based on circulating levels of vitamins and the appearance of characteristic deficiency symptoms, there seems to be an increased requirement for certain vitamins (vitamin B_6, folacin, vitamin C, vitamin B_{12}, and possibly vitamin E) (2).

Television advertising would have us believe in the need for vitamin supplements to maintain health and vitality even though we may be eating a good diet. The rationale for this belief is that vitamin supplements are "insurance" in case vitamins are not present—or are present in insufficient amounts—in the food we eat. Actually vitamin supplements are not necessary for most people. The myth that depleted soils yield products with inadequate nutrients is indeed a myth. Modern methods of food technology, which include crop rotation, soil tests, and routine enrichment of soils, together with analysis of crops, ensure that the products are nutritionally adequate. It must also be remembered that the major nutrients of plant foods, protein, fat, carbohydrate, vitamins, and fiber, are determined by the genetic structure of the plant. Minor differences in mineral content may reflect the mineral elements in the soil. The best way to ensure an adequate intake of the required nutrients still is to eat a balanced diet with foods selected from the four major food groups—dairy products, meat, fruits and vegetables, and bread and cereals. And luckily many different dietary patterns can supply the required nutrients in adequate amounts.

However, it is much more appealing to believe that the illnesses that still plague mankind are due to vitamin shortages which can easily be corrected by the "right" supplements. Much of the belief in the curative powers of vitamin supplements is the result of misinterpretation of research with animals. Take, for example, the curious case of vitamin E. The conditions said to be cured by or treatable with vitamin E range from acne and other skin diseases to varicose veins and all types of vascular diseases and include practically all noninfectious diseases that have been described. In healthy individuals it is supposed to enhance sexual potency, especially in men, prevent heart attacks, and slow down the aging process.

Now let us consider the facts. Since the best way to learn about a nutrient is to study the effects of its deficiency in animal systems, it was soon discovered that vitamin E deficiency in rats leads to reproductive failure and fetal resorption in the female and testicular degeneration in the male. Normal reproduction performance in rats is maintained by approximately 1 mg of alpha-tocopherol per animal per day and excess supplementation does not result in superior performances by either sex. With overpopulation rather than underpopulation a problem in today's world, claims of marginal vitamin E intakes and the need for supplementation seem unsubstantiated.

A nutritional muscular dystrophy which responds to treatment with vitamin E can be induced in animals placed on vitamin E-deficient diets. As a result, vitamin E determinations have been made on, and supplementation with large amounts of vitamin E has been tried in, patients with muscular dystrophy. These patients were not found to have low serum tocopherol levels, nor was vitamin E therapy at all effective.

Vitamin E-deficient ruminants and rabbits, but not primates, develop a cardiac necrosis and fibrosis which led inevitably to claims for vitamin E supplements as therapy for patients with coronary disease (3). Unfortunately, scientific research does not support the claims of the enthusiasts (4). Some scientists (5, 6), however, do report an improvement in intermittent claudication, as demonstrated by improved walking distance, in patients given vitamin E supplements, although others do not (7, 8).

Other claims that have been made for supplemental vitamin E, such as a delay in onset of aging symptoms, protection against smog, prevention of wrinkles, alleviation of scar tissue, and therapy for cancer all need further research, evaluation, and substantiation.

Vitamin E deficiency is rare in humans. First, vitamin E is widely distributed in foods—especially vegetable oils and products made from oils, as well as vegetables and whole grains. Second, a considerable amount of vitamin E is stored in tissues and an extended period of time is needed to deplete the stores before vitamin deficiency can occur. Actually, there is only one long-term study (9) in which attempts were made to study vitamin E deficiency in humans. After three years on a diet low in vitamin E, plasma tocopherol levels of hospitalized men were sharply decreased. There was a slight decrease in the life span of red blood cells, and an increase in the susceptibility of the red blood cell to *in vitro* hemolysis in hydrogen peroxide (a test that is used to estimate vitamin E deficiency). There were no other manifestations of disease.

Are there individuals or populations who require vitamin E supplements? Premature infants whose vitamin E stores are low may develop a hemolytic anemia if not supplemented at birth with vitamin E. Persons who have difficulties with fat absorption, children and young adults with cystic fibrosis, and patients with steatorrhea, may also develop vitamin E deficiency as manifested by low blood levels of this vitamin, although no disease attributable to vitamin E deficiency has been reported in these subjects. Recent reports (10–12) also indicate that the vitamin E requirement is increased when the polyunsaturated fatty acid content of the diet is elevated, since vitamin E is an antioxidant and protects polyunsaturated fatty acids against oxidation. Luckily both of these nutrients occur together in foods.

Toxicity studies of large dietary doses of vitamin E have only recently been reported. Animal studies reveal depressed growth, interference with thyroid function, increased requirements for vitamin D and K, and elevated lipid and cholesterol levels in liver (13, 14). In humans, supplements of vitamin E above 400 IU per day revealed minor complaints of nausea, intestinal distress, fatigue, flulike symptoms, and a variety of nonspecific complaints (15, 16). In general, for most individuals daily doses below 300 IU have caused no problems. However, it should be noted that the 1974 RDA for women is 12 IU.

VITAMIN C

Most species of animals are able to synthesize their own vitamin C. Only a few—the guinea pig, the Indian fruit-eating bat, certain birds, primates, and man—have evidently lost the enzyme systems that convert precursors to ascorbic acid. Yet all species of animals require vitamin C. The question is how much vitamin C do humans require. If need is based on what animals eat in their natural habitat, the gorilla eats vegetation that provides 4.5 g of vitamin C per day and this figure suggests an intake of 1 to 2 g for humans. If it is based on the amount synthesized by the rat, when extrapolated to man, a figure of 1.8 to 4.1 g is obtained. However, although nutritional experiments on humans are few and expensive, experiments with human volunteers on low vitamin C diets showed that as little as 10 mg of vitamin C/subject/day could prevent or cure scurvy, the vitamin C deficiency disease (17, 18). Ascorbic acid at a level of 30 mg/day replaced the body pool—the amount of vitamin C turned over each day (19). The 1974 RDA for vitamin C is 45 mg for both men and women.

Vitamin C has many uses in the body. It acts in oxidation-reduction reactions in the body; it participates in collagen formation, tissue regeneration, and bone deposition, in the conversion of folic acid to its active form, folinic acid, in the metabolism of certain amino acids, and in other biological systems such as steroid transformations in the adrenal gland. Moreover, reports are available to indicate that vitamin C deficiency in guinea pigs contributes to hypercholesterolemia and an increased level of cholesterol in liver (20, 21). Other reports indicated that the long-term administration of ascorbic acid prevents experimentally induced atherosclerosis in rats, rabbits, and guinea pigs (22, 23).

Although from these reports elevated levels of ascorbic acid seem to have a role in clinical atherosclerosis, more recent publications link excessive ascorbic acid supplements to hypercholesterolemia in rats (24) and in atherosclerotic humans (25). The true involvement of ascorbic acid in atherogenesis awaits confirmation.

By far the most popular claim for vitamin C supplements is in connection with the common cold. In the book *Vitamin C and the Common Cold*, Dr. Linus Pauling, himself a vitamin C enthusiast, cites the results of several studies to indicate that vitamin C in large doses can prevent or ameliorate the common cold. On closer examination of the data included in the book, the significance of some of the results is highly questionable. In some cases the studies were not double blind; in others differences between control and experimental groups were too small for meaningful comparisons; other reports were subjective discourses with no data presented. Some of the more recent interesting results include those of Wilson and Loh (26), who gave 500 mg tablets of vitamin C to one group of school children in Ireland and a placebo to another group. They reported that vitamin C significantly reduced "the severity and total intensity of colds in girls, but does not benefit cold symptoms in boys." This, I believe, is the first report of a sex difference in the use of vitamin C.

In the previous year, a group of researchers in Canada (27) had performed a double-blind study on vitamin C and the common cold and reported that the vitamin C-supplemented group had 30% fewer days of disability than the unsupplemented group.

Further studies by this group (28) indicate that, although there are few adequately controlled clinical trials, under certain circumstances an increased intake of vitamin C may reduce the *severity*—not the incidence—of upper respiratory infections in those persons whose tissues are not already fully saturated. However, increasing the daily dose above what is necessary to produce tissue saturation provides no significant benefit. It must be mentioned that during an upper respiratory infection (and possible other stress situations as well), a higher intake than normal of vitamin C may be required to maintain tissue saturation. It should be noted that in a study with a limited number of predominantly well-nourished individuals who had colds, in whom there was a reduction of sickness experience associated with large doses of vitamin C, the same alleviation of symptoms was observed over a wide range of vitamin C intake—from 250 mg to 2 g per day (28). In general, the use of vitamin C to *prevent* colds seems without justification at this time.

However, the benefit of large supplements of vitamin C in cold *therapy* rather than prevention still requires confirmation and evaluation. In the meantime, the use of megavitamin C must be approached with caution. Large doses may not be for everybody. In spite of the fact that vitamin C is a water-soluble vitamin and excesses beyond those which yield tissue saturation are theoretically excreted, side effects have been reported. Large doses of vitamin C may cause diarrhoea, very acid urines, and kidney and bladder stones in animals. Excess vitamin C may interfere with the action of certain drugs. In a report in the Russian literature, 6 g of ascorbic acid given to 20 pregnant women for three successive days caused abortions in 16.

More recently two New York physicians observed that some patients who were taking 1 g of vitamin C daily had extremely low levels of vitamin B_{12}

in blood (29). If this is continued it might result in pernicious anemia and irreversible destruction of the spinal cord. When food is ingested with large amounts of vitamin C, vitamin B_{12} is actually destroyed. Therefore, the authors concluded that it would be very unwise to take more than 0.5 g of ascorbic acid without regular evaluation of the vitamin B_{12} status.

Furthermore, guinea pigs fed high levels of ascorbic acid during the last half of pregnancy produced pups which exhibited a higher ascorbic acid catabolism during the first 10 days of life than the controls. When these animals were placed on an ascorbic acid deficient diet, they developed scurvy four days earlier than the young from a control group and they died seven days sooner than the control animals (30). This may be an indication that the organism adapts to higher levels of ascorbic acid with higher requirement thereafter.

It must be remembered that vitamins are potent chemical compounds which exhibit their biological effects in microgram quantities. Some of them (vitamins A and D) have already been proven to be toxic in large doses. The indiscriminate use of large doses of vitamins should be discouraged.

REFERENCES

1. Aftergood, L., Alexander, A. R., and Alfin-Slater, R. B. *Nutrition Reports International* **11**:295 (1975).
2. Oral Contraceptives and Nutrition, Statement by Food and Nutrition Board, National Research Council, National Academy of Sciences (1975).
3. Shute, W. E. and Taub, H. J. *Vitamin E for Ailing and Healthy Hearts*, Pyramid House (1969).
4. Rinzler, S. H., Bakst, H., Benjamin, Z. H., Bob, A. L., and Travell, J. *Circulation* **1**:288 (1950).
5. Boyd, A. M., Ratcliffe, A. H., Jepson, R. B., and James, G. W. H. *J. Bone Joint Surg.* **31–B**:225 (1949).
6. Haeger, K. *Actuelle Therapie* **3**:108 (1973).
7. Baer, S. and Heine, W. I. *J.A.M.A.* **139**:733 (1949).
8. Hamilton, M., Wilson, G. M., Armitage, P., and Boyd, J. T. *Lancet* **1**:367 (1953).
9. Horwitt, M. K. *Am. J. Clin. Nutr.* **8**:451 (1960).
10. Harris, P. L. and Embree, N. D. *Am. J. Clin. Nutr.* **13**:385 (1963).
11. Jager, F. C. *Ann. N.Y. Acad. Sci.* **203**:199 (1972).
12. Alfin-Slater, R. B., Wells, P., Aftergood, L., and Melnick, D. *J. Am. Oil Chemists Soc.* **50**:479 (1973).
13. March, B. E., Wong, E., Seier, L., Sim, J., and Biely, J. *J. Nutrition* **103**:371 (1973).
14. Alfin-Slater, R. B., Aftergood, L., and Kishineff, S. Tenth International Congress of Nutrition 191 (1972) Abstract.

15. Vogelsang, A. B., Shute, E. V., and Shute, W. E. *Med. Record* **160**:279 (1947).
16. King, R. A. *J. Bone Joint Surg.* **31B**:443 (1949).
17. Baker, E. M., Hodges, R. E., Hood, J., Sauberlich, H. E., and March, S. C. *Am. J. Clin. Nutr.* **22**:549 (1969).
18. Hodges, R. E., Baker, E. M., Hood, J., Sauberlich, H. E., and March, S. C. *Am. J. Clin. Nutr.* **22**:535 (1969).
19. Baker, E. M. *Am. J. Clin. Nutr.* **20**:583 (1967).
20. Ginter, E., Babala, J., and Cerven, J. *J. Atheroscler. Res.* **10**:341 (1969).
21. Ginter, E., Ondreicka, R., Bobek, P., and Sinko, V. *J. Nutr.* **97**:261 (1969).
22. Sokoloff, B., Hori, M., Saelhof, C. C., Wrzolek R., and Imai, T. *J. Am. Geriat. Soc.* **14**:1239 (1966).
23. Sokoloff, B., Hori, M., Saelhof, C. C., McConnell, B., and Imai, T. *J. Nutr.* **91**: 107 (1967).
24. Klevay, L. A. *Fed. Proc.* **34**:899 (1975).
25. Spittle, C. R. *Lancet* **2**:1280 (1971).
26. Wilson, C. W. M. and Loh, H. S. *Lancet*, 638 (1973).
27. Anderson, T. W., Reid, R. B. W., and Beaton, G. H. *Canad. Med. Assn. J.* **107**: 503 (1972).
28. Anderson, T. W. Western Hemisphere Nutrition Congress IV. Abstracts p. 67 (1974).
29. Herbert, V. and Jacob, E. *J.A.M.A.* **230**:241 (1974).
30. Norkus, E. and Rosso, P. *Fed. Proceedings* **34**:884 (1975). Abstract.

8

The Osteoporosis Problem

LOUIS V. AVIOLI, M.D.

Department of Medicine, Washington University School of Medicine, St. Louis, Missouri

Osteoporosis of the senile or postmenopausal variety is defined as a skeletal disorder in which the absolute amount of bone is decreased relative to that of younger or menstruating individuals although the remaining bone is normal in chemical composition. Symptomatic senile or postmenopausal osteoporosis syndromes are classically considered to result from the universal loss of bone that normally attends senescence in both sexes and begins in the third or fourth decade of life. Although comparable decrements in the functional capacity of the heart, lungs, kidney, and nervous tissue (i.e., nerve conduction time) also attend the aging process, the decrease in bone mass may lead to significant incapacitation and result in fractures and immobilization in the aged individual not only requiring significant hospitalization time but often resulting in relative inactivity.

This is a problem of considerable magnitude: approximately 6.3 million people in the United States are currently suffering from acute problems related to weakened vertebral bones. Perhaps even more significant is the fact that 8 million Americans today have *chronic* problems related to the spine compared with 6 million reported in 1963. Moreover, recent epidemiological surveys indicate that a minimum of 10% of the female population over 50 years of age suffers from bone loss severe enough to cause hip, vertebrae, or long-bone fractures; surveys performed in homes for the aged and of ambulatory individuals 50 to 95 years of age requiring medical care also disclosed symptomatic (i.e., back pain) osteoporosis in 15 and 50% of these populations, respectively.

The consequences of osteoporosis are magnified in the postmenopausal female, resulting in major orthopedic problems in approximately 25 to 30% of postmenopausal women. The incidence of symptomatic osteoporosis appears to be four times greater in women than in men.

Although the total female population in the United States tripled from 31 million in 1900 to 91 million in 1960, the total annual number of vertebral or hip fractures rose from 11,000 to 62,000. The rise in fracture rate was twice as fast as the population gain because of the disproportionate increment in the number of aged females susceptible to fractures of the hip and vertebral column. It should also be emphasized that demographic data indicate that the over 50 age group is the fastest growing minority in the United States and that of the one million (approximate) fractures experienced each year by women aged 45 years or older in the United States, about 700,000 are incurred by women with osteoporosis. In 1968, falls were the leading cause of nontransport accidental deaths in all persons and the leading cause of all accidental deaths in elderly white females in the United States. Approximately three-quarters of all deaths from falls occur in patients aged 65 and over, with a female:male fracture incidence ratio of 8:1. The rate (per 1000 population per year) of hip fractures in white women due to minimal trauma increases from 2.0 at ages 50 to 64, to 5.0 at ages 65 to 74, to 10 at ages greater than 75 years.

Although the ravages of the relentless decrease in bone mass are well known, the reason for this age-related skeletal loss is still purely conjectural at best. Dietary indiscretion, inactivity, decrease in muscle mass, hormonal imbalance, renal dysfunction leading either to inability to conserve calcium or to secondary increments in circulating hormones which resorb bone (i.e., parathyroid hormone), and acquired defects in intestinal absorption of nutrients essential for "bone health" have also been implicated as causative factors. Accordingly, therapeutic regimens emphasizing the need for adequate calcium intake, muscular tone and activity, dietary vitamin D or C or adequate sunlight exposure, estrogens (in the postmenopausal or early-castrated female) and agents which supposedly "strengthen" bones, such as sodium flouride, have all been advocated. To date, the results of these so-called therapeutic measures have resulted in limited if any overall symptomatic improvement in skeletal pains or in the fracture incidence in the aged population at risk. Limited observations in females treated following cessation of menses (2 to 3 years after menopause) suggest that short-term estrogen replacement therapy (9 to 14 months) may prove beneficial in decreasing the accelerated rate of bone loss of the appendicular skeleton (forearm and fingers) although more prolonged therapy may prove detrimental in this regard. Dietary surveys often reveal relative calcium and vitamin D deficiences and high phosphate intakes in symptomatic osteoporotic females, but to date the preventative therapeutic benefit of well-balanced dietary regimens in reversing the disease process and fracture incidence in these same subjects has not been established.

BIBLIOGRAPHY

Aaron, J. E., Stasiak, L., Gallagher, J. C., Longton, E. B., Nicholson, M., Anderson, J., and Nordin, B. E. C. Frequency of Osteomalacia and Osteoporosis in Fractures of the Proximal Femur. *Lancet* **1**:7851 (1974).

Aaron, J. E., Gallagher, J. C., and Nordin, B. E. C. Seasonal Variation of Histological Osteomalacia in Femoral Neck Fractures. *Lancet* **2**:84 (1974).

Ackerman, P. G. and Toro, G. Calcium Balance in Elderly Women. *J. Gerontol.* **9**:446 (1954).

Adams, P., Davies, G. T., and Sweetman, P. Osteoporosis and the Effects of Aging on Bone Mass in Elderly Men and Women. *Quart. J. Med.* **39**:601 (1970).

Aitken, J. M., Anderson, J. B., and Horton, P. W. Seasonal Variations in Bone Mineral Content after the Menopause. *Nature* **241**:59 (1973).

Aitken, J. M., Hart, D. M., and Lindsay, R. Oestrogen Replacement Therapy for Prevention of Osteoporosis after Oophorectomy. *Brit. Med. J.* **2**:515 (1973).

Alevizaki, C. C., Ikkos, D. G., and Singhelakis, P. Progressive Decrease of True Intestinal Calcium Absorption with Age in Normal Man. *J. Nuc. Med.* **14**:760 (1973).

Alhava, E. M. and Puittinen, J. Fractures of the Upper End of the Femur as an Index of Senile Osteoporosis in Finland. *Ann. Clin. Res.* **5**:398 (1973).

Atkinson, P. J. Variation in Trabecular Structure of Vertebrae with Age. *Calc. Tiss. Res.* 1:24 (1967).

Baker, P. T. and Agnel, J. L. Old Age Changes in Bone Density: Sex and Race Factors in the United States. *Human Biol.* **37**:104 (1965).

Boukhris, R. and Becker, K. L. The Inter-relationship between Vertebral Fractures and Osteoporosis. *Clin. Orthop. Res.* **90**:209 (1973).

Boukhris, R. and Becker, K. L. Schmorl's Nodes and Osteoporosis. *Clin. Orthop. Rel. Res.* **104**:275 (1974).

Bullamore, J. R., Wilkinson, R., Gallagher, J. C., Nordin, B. E. C., and Marshall, D. H. Effect of Age on Calcium Absorption. *Lancet* **2**:535 (1970).

Cohen, M. B. and Rubini, M. E. The Treatment of Osteoporosis with Sodium Fluoride. *Clin. Orthop. Rel. Res.* **40**:147 (1965).

Cohn, S. G., Dombrowski, C. S., Hauser, W., and Atkins, H. L. High Calcium Diet and the Parameters of Calcium Metabolism in Osteoporosis. *Am. J. Clin. Nutr.* **21**:1246 (1968).

Cohn, S. G., Dombrowski, C. S., Hauser, W., Klopper, J. and Atkins, H. L.: Effects of Porcine Calcitonin on Calcium Metabolism in Osteoporosis. *J. Clin. Endocr.* **33**:719 (1971).

Conacher, W. D. H. Metabolic Bone Disease in the Elderly. *Practitioner* **210**:351 (1973).

Corless, D., Boucher, B. J., Beer, M., Gupta, S. P., and Cohen, R. D. Vitamin D Status in Long-Stay Geriatric Patients. *Lancet* **1**:1404 (1975).

Dalen, N., Lamke, B., and Wallgren, A. Bone-Mineral Losses in Oophorectomized Women. *J. Bone Joint Surg.* **56A**:1235 (1974).

Dallas, I. and Nordin, B. E. C. The Relation Between Calcium Intake and Roentgenologic Osteoporosis. *Am. J. Clin. Nutr.* **11**:263 (1962).

Davis, E. M., Lanzl, L. H., and Cox, A. B. Detection, Prevention and Retardation of Menopausal Osteoporosis. *J. Obstet. Gynec.* **36**:187 (1970).

Dudl, R. J., Ensinck, J. W., Bayling, D., Chesnut, C. H., Sherrard, D., and Nelp, W. B. Evaluation of Intravenous Calcium as Therapy for Osteoporosis. *Am. J. Med.* **55**:631 (1973).

Ellis, F. R., Holesh, S. and Ellis, J. W. Incidence of Osteoporosis in Vegetarians and Omnivores. *Am. J. Clin. Nutr.* **25**:555 (1972).

Exton-Smith, A. N. and Stewart, R. J. C. Bone Resorption in Old Age. *Proc. Roy. Soc. Med.* **65**:14 (1972).

Exton-Smith, A. N., Millard, P. H., Payne, P. R., and Wheeler, E. F. Pattern of Development and Loss of Bone with Age. *Lancet* **2**:1154 (1969).

Franke, J., Rempel, H., and Franke, M. Three Years Experience with Sodium Fluoride Therapy of Osteoporosis. *Acta. Orthop. Scand.* **45**:1 (1974).

Garn, S. M. Calcium Requirements for Bone Buildings and Skeletal Maintenance. *Am. J. Clin. Nutr.* **23**:1149 (1970).

Garn, S. M. The Course of Bone Gain and the Phases of Bone Loss. *Orthop. Clin. N. Am.* **3**:503 (1972).

Garn, S. M., Rohmann, C. A., and Wagner, B. Bone Loss as a General Phenomenon in Man. *Fed. Proc.* **26**:1729 (1967).

Goldsmith, M. F., Johnston, J. O., Ury, H., Vose, G., and Colbert, C. Bone Mineral Estimation in Normal and Osteoporotic Women. *J. Bone Joint Surg.* **53A**:83 (1971).

Herberg, C. A. Treatment of Postmenopausal Osteoporosis with Estrogens and Androgens. *Acta Endocrinol.* **34**:51 (1960).

Hurxthal, L. M. and Vose, G. P. The Relationship of Dietary Calcium Intake to Radiographic Bone Density in Normal and Osteoporotic Persons. *Calc. Tiss. Res.* **4**:245 (1969).

Inkovaara, J., Heikinheimo, R., Jarvinen, K., Kasurinen, U., Hanhijarvi, H., and Iisalo, E. Prophylactic Fluoride Treatment and Aged Bones. *Brit. Med. J.* **3**:73 (1975).

Iskrant, A. P. The Etiology of Fractured Hips in Females: A Study of Suspected Relationships Between Osteoporosis and Fractures from Falls. *Am. J. Pub. Health* **58**:485 (1975).

Jowsey, J., Riggs, B., Kelly, P. J., and Hoffman, D. L. Effect of Combined Therapy with Sodium Fluoride, Vitamin D and Calcium in Osteoporosis. *Am. J. Med.* **54**:43 (1972).

Jurist, J. M. *In Vivo* Determination of the Elastic Response of Bone II. Ulnar Resonant Frequency in Osteoporotic, Diabetic and Normal Subjects. *Phys. Med. Biol.* **15**:427 (1970).

Lachman, E. Osteoporosis: The Potentialities and Limitations of its Roentgenologic Diagnosis. *Am. J. Roentgenol.* **74**:712 (1955).

Lutwak, L. Symposium on Osteoporosis: Nutritional Aspects of Osteoporosis. *J. Am. Geriat. Soc.* **17**:115 (1969).

Meema, H. E. Cortical Bone Atrophy and Osteoporosis as a Manifestation of Aging. *Am. J. Roentgen.* **89**:1287 (1963).

Meema, H. E. and Meema, S. Prevention of Postmenopausal Osteoporosis by Hormone Treatment of the Menopause. *Can. Med. Assn. J.* **99**:248 (1968).

Melick, R. A. and Baird, C. W. The Effect of 'Parenabol' on Patients with Osteoporosis. *Med. J. Australia* **2**:960 (1970).

Miller, R. G. The Treatment of Osteoporosis—A Report of a Double Blind Therapeutic Trial. *Gerontol. Clin.* **11**:244 (1969).

Newton-John, H. F. and Morgan, D. B. The Loss of Bone with Age, Osteoporosis and Fractures. *Clin. Orthop. Rel. Res.* **71**:229 (1970).

Nilsson, B. E. and Westlin, N. E. Changes in Bone Mass in Alcoholics. *Clin. Orthop. Rel. Res.* **90**:229 (1973).

Riggs, B. L., Jowsey, J., Kelly, P. J., Jones, J. D., and Maher, F. T. Effect of Sex Hormone on Bone in Primary Osteoporosis. *J. Clin. Invest.* **48**:1065 (1969).

Riggs, B. L., Jowsey, J., Goldsmith, R. S., Kelly, P. S., Hoffman, D. L., and Arnaud, C. D. Short- and Long-Term Effects of Estrogen and Synthetic Anabolic Hormone in Postmenopausal Osteoporosis. *J. Clin. Invest.* **51**:1659 (1972).

Saville, P. D. Symptomatic Osteoporosis and the Menopause. *Clin. Orthop. Rel. Res.* **55**:43 (1967).

Smith, R. W., Jr., Eyler, W. R., and Mellinger, R. C. On the Incidence of Senile Osteoporosis. *Ann. Int. Med.* **52**:773 (1960).

Smith, D. M., Khairi, M. R. A., and Johnston, C. C., Jr. The Loss of Bone Mineral with Aging and its Relationship to Risk of Fracture. *J. Clin. Invest.* **56**:311 (1975).

Thomas, T. G. and Stevens, R. S. Social Effects of Fractures of the Neck of the Femur. *Brit. Med. J.* **3**:456 (1974).

Wachman, A. and Bernstein, D. S. Diet and Osteoporosis. *Lancet* **1**:958 (1968).

Walker, A. R. P. The Human Requirement of Calcium: Should Low Intakes be Supplemented? *Am. J. Clin. Nutr.* **25**:518 (1972).

PART 4

Obesity

9

Hunger and Satiety in Man

SAMI A. HASHIM, M.D.

Department of Medicine, St. Luke's Hospital Center and Institute of Human Nutrition, College of Physicians and Surgeons, Columbia University, New York, New York

The study of food intake in man has not kept pace with our understanding of food intake behavior in experimental animals. It is becoming increasingly evident, however, that regulation of energy balance in normal man is a physiologic phenomenon. First, the common observation has been made that many adults maintain a stable body weight between postadolescence and age 40 years, and that some people appear to maintain body weight within narrow ranges throughout a life span of 70 or more years (1, 2). Second, it has been shown that within limits, an increase in physical activity is associated with an increase in food intake without a corresponding increase in body weight. However, paradoxically, man has the capability of increasing his food intake while engaging in occupations of increasing sedentariness, with consequences of increasing his body stores of fat (3). Thus, in our society the executive who is leading a sedentary life may consume as many calories per day as the person engaged in heavy physical work. Similar observations have been made in sedentary and exercising animals (4).

An important concept has emerged that under normal circumstances man, like other animals, regulates food intake to meet energy expenditure. In this manner, body weight is kept within a narrow range for many years. Such a regulation of energy balance may not be precise in some individuals since fat, as a proportion of body weight, increases with age, at the expense of lean body mass (5, 6). Recent studies of experimental obesity in man indicate that

Supported in part by grant (AM-17624) from the National Institutes of Health.

when volunteers agreed to overfeed themselves, body weight (and body fat) increased during the time of overeating. When the subjects returned to their usual self-selected diets, their food intake diminished and their body weight returned within a few weeks to its level prior to voluntary gorging (7, 8). Similarly, rats made obese by force feeding diminished their food intake and lost weight down to the level pior to force feeding once the animals were allowed to eat spontaneously (9). These studies provide support for the concept that maintenance of body weight occurs by regulation of energy balance. Hence adjustments and adaptations must occur in food intake and energy expenditure of persons who maintain body weight within narrow ranges throughout their life span. Conversely, those who do not achieve such a regulation succumb either to a cachexia or obesity. In fact, obesity is far more common that cachexia. Approximately 25% of men and women in the United States between the ages of 30 and 39 years exceed the "best" weight by 20% or more. The proportions for men and women, respectively, rise to 32% and 40% between ages 40 and 49 years and to 34% and 46% between ages 50 and 59 years. Thus, we are living in an age of anxiety with regard to our energy balance, caloric intake, and nutritional status (Fig. 1).

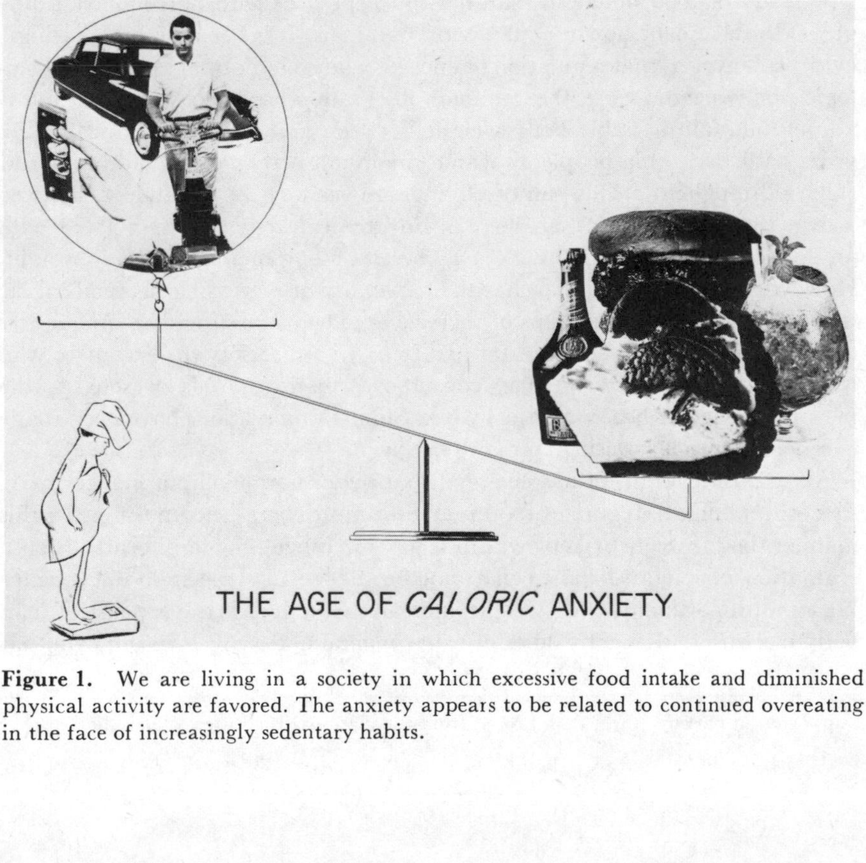

Figure 1. We are living in a society in which excessive food intake and diminished physical activity are favored. The anxiety appears to be related to continued overeating in the face of increasingly sedentary habits.

FOOD INTAKE IN MAN

Despite the clear evidence for regulation of energy balance in man, a striking proportion of our population develops obesity. Such a disorder can be viewed as a disturbance in energy balance. One side of the equation is food intake. Recent developments in this area indicate that the obese persons is one in whom food intake regulation in relation to energy expenditure is disturbed. Moreover, there is evidence to indicate that such a disturbance is related to factors in the environment that eventually provide "force feeding" opportunities without regard to the physiological demands of the individual.

Food intake occurs in response to a desire for food (hunger) and stops in response to lack of such desire for food (satiety). Usually the duration of satiety is longer than that of hunger. Thus food, the "curative" agent for hunger, is selected in the belief that it helps restore or maintain health. Such a belief is often true in a society where serious malnutrition does not occur when food is readily available and easily procurable. However, under these circumstances, the "hazard" exists that the individual may eat and overeat not only for nutritional purposes, but for other reasons as well. In recent years the behavioral sciences have made some important observations with regard to eating behavior in man that have improved our understanding of the pathogenesis of overeating.

There are two basic views about reasons for overeating (10). One proposition is that food intake is increased because of subtle metabolic derangement affecting signals transmitted to the food regulatory or satiety center, or that the sensitivity threshold of the center to the signals is altered. Thus, food is "pulled" into the body at an enhanced rate or in larger quantity, resulting in disruption of energy balance and consequent obesity. The second proposition is that food intake is increased because of force feeding in response to external factors in the environment that are nonphysiological. Thus, food is "pushed" into the body, resulting easily in an intake that is in excess of energy expenditure. Whereas a whole variety of metabolic and endocrine factors appear to play a role in food intake (11, 12), a primary lesion responsible for overeating in the face of nonchanging or even diminished physical activity has not been identified. When the individual is already obese, certain metabolic disorders may appear, such as hyperlipidemia, diabetes, basal hyperinsulinism, and hypertension. However, such disorders have been shown to disappear or diminish in intensity after a substantial reduction in body weight has occurred. In contrast, certain determinants of eating behavior have been identified as environmental influences on the individual that result in overeating. The prevalence of such external influences on eating is widespread in our society, so that a substantial proportion of our population appears to succumb to them. In essence, the external determinants of eating induce overeating in certain individuals in whom the internal physiologic mechanisms are overridden. The net effect is force feeding. Thus, a reversal of overeating to energy intake commensurate with energy expenditure must involve "de-externalization" and therefore a change in food intake behavior (13, 14).

EXTERNALITY AND INTERNALITY

In 1964, Stunkard and Koch (15) conducted a study of gastric contractions in lean and obese subjects and correlated them with self-reports of hunger. In the fasting state the subjects swallowed a gastric balloon, and their gastric contractions were recorded continuously for the ensuing four hours. At 15-minute intervals each subject was asked, "Do you feel hungry?" to which the answer was "yes" or "no." In this manner, a record was obtained of gastric contractions which coincided with the presence or absence of hunger. In the lean subjects, there was a positive correlation between gastric contractions and reports of hunger. However, in the obese subjects there was no such correlation. Thus, with respect to one bodily parameter usually associated with hunger, the obese appears to be out of phase with the subjective feeling of hunger. Pursuing this lead, Schachter and his graduate students have conducted a series of experiments in normal and obese subjects which have provided strong support to the concept that obese persons, in contrast to lean individuals, are relatively insensitive to "internal" cues for hunger and satiety and are more responsive to "external" food-relevant cues. In support of this hypothesis, Schachter and his associates proceeded to manipulate a variety of bodily states in their subjects while observing their food intake behavior. An example of such manipulation was food deprivation (16). Normal and obese subjects had either full stomachs (in response to recent ingestion of roast beef sandwiches) or empty stomachs prior to the experimental eating situation. Each subject remained unaware of the real purpose of the experiment through some plausible explanation. Lean and obese subjects with full or empty stomachs were asked to sample crackers of differing tastes and rate them on a long set of rating scales with respect to their taste during a period of 15 minutes. The subjects, of course, remained unaware that they were being observed through a one-way mirror, which formed the "wall" between the room where they were engaged in their taste tasks and the observation room. As predicted, the normal subjects ate considerably fewer crackers when their stomachs were full than when their stomachs were empty. In contrast, the obese subjects ate as many crackers when their stomachs were full as when they were empty. Manipulation of another bodily state, fear (associated with inhibition of gastric motility and rise in blood sugar), had no effect on the amount of crackers eaten by the obese subjects, but had a striking effect on the amount eaten by normal subjects (16, 17).

The same group went on to investigate the effect of manipulating external factors relevant to the food itself on food intake behavior of lean and obese subjects. These included quantity, saliency, and taste. In response to the sight of varying quantities of food, obese subjects ate significantly more than normals when presented with an abundance of food, and ate significantly less than normals when presented with a scarcity of food (18). In response to manipulation of saliency, obese subjects ate significantly more food than normals when the food was highly visible and significantly less when the food was dimly in sight (19). When food taste was manipulated, obese subjects drank more than normals when the milk shake was flavored pleasantly and considerably less than normals when the milk shake was adulterated with quinine (20). Differences in other aspects of food intake behavior were found between obese and normal subjects. These included the amount of food eaten ad libitum (more for the obese), the amount of food consumed per meal (more for the obese), the frequency of meals (more frequent for the obese), the rate of eating (faster for the obese), and work and eating. When food was easily accessible, obese subjects ate more than normals; when food was hard to get at, obese subjects ate less than normals. These studies were summarized by Schachter and Schachter and Rodin in recent reviews (21, 22). The conclusion is that obese persons are under external rather than internal controls with regard to eating. The obese are more likely to eat and eat more than lean individuals when food-relevant cues are present and salient. In contrast, when food-relevant cues are absent or low in saliency, the obese are less likely to eat, or likely to eat less than normals.

THE FEEDING MACHINE

Our group has conducted a series of studies of food intake behavior in obese and lean subjects hospitalized for weeks on the metabolic ward during which time the subjects ingest their food spontaneously from an automatically monitored food dispensing apparatus. We have applied certain features of the operant conditioning technique previously used in experimental animals (23–25) for the study of food intake in man. Initially, we constructed a feeding machine (26) that would allow the subject to feed himself spontaneously a liquid formula diet delivered through a mouthpiece at the command of a button. The feeding machine (Fig. 2) consists of a refrigerator in which a reservoir of formula diet is placed on top of a magnetic stirrer (bottom shelf of refrigerator) which serves to keep the formula diet homogeneous. A syringe

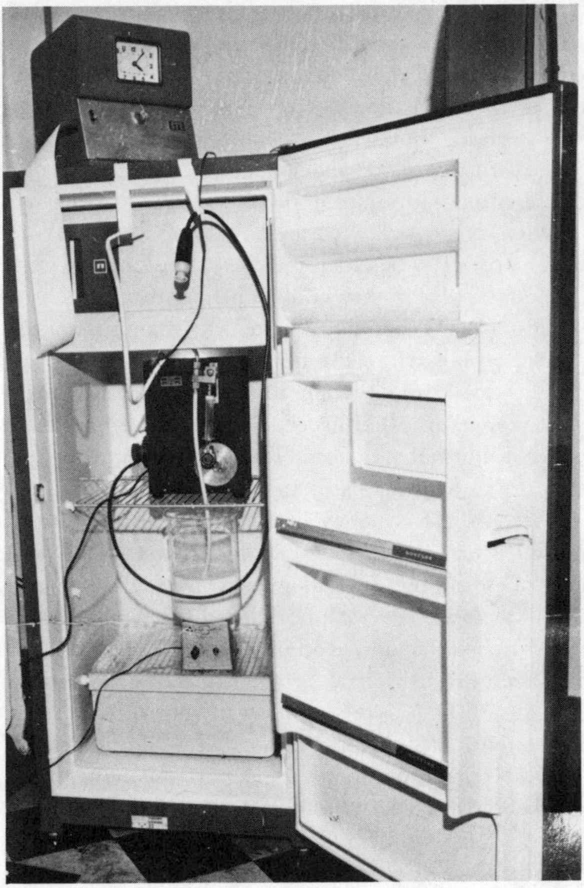

Figure 2. Automatically monitored food dispensing machine. The refrigerated liquid formula diet, constantly stirred, is delived by the syringe pump in a predetermined amount upon activation of a button. The event is recorded by a printing timer which, in actual use, is remote from the subject.

pump (second shelf) is connected by one flexible tube to the formula reservoir and by another tube to a mouthpiece. Upon activation of an electric button, a predetermined amount of formula is delivered directly into the mouth. The amount of formula thus delivered can be varied, but a fixed volume was selected (7 ml) as a "comfortable" mouthful. Thus, one button push delivers 7 ml and the machine can keep up with the subject as often as he or she chooses to push the button. Unbeknown to the subject, the button-pushing is automatically monitored by a switch placed in the path of the rotating disc of the syringe pump. This switch activates a timer which for illustrative purposes is placed on top of the refrigerator. In actual use, the timer is located in another room and the subject remains unaware that every time the button is pushed, the event, giving the exact time of day to the minute, is recorded. The timer also prints button pushing within the minute. Thus, if the subject chooses to eat (drink) many times during one minute, the record clearly will reveal the activity. In this way details of button pushing reflect food intake continuously on a 24-hour basis.

The subject "lives" with the machine, which is placed near the bed. In actual use the reservoir and pump mechanism are concealed from the subject. All that needs to be done by the subject is to ensure that the mouthpiece is in the mouth and the button to activate the system is in the hand (Fig. 3). The subject is asked to choose one flavor of formula (vanilla, chocolate, etc.) which will remain the same throughout the study. The formula itself is a complete diet providing 50% of the calories from carbohydrate, 20% from protein, and 30% from fat, and contains adequate amounts of vitamins and minerals. Privacy of the subject with the machine is ensured.

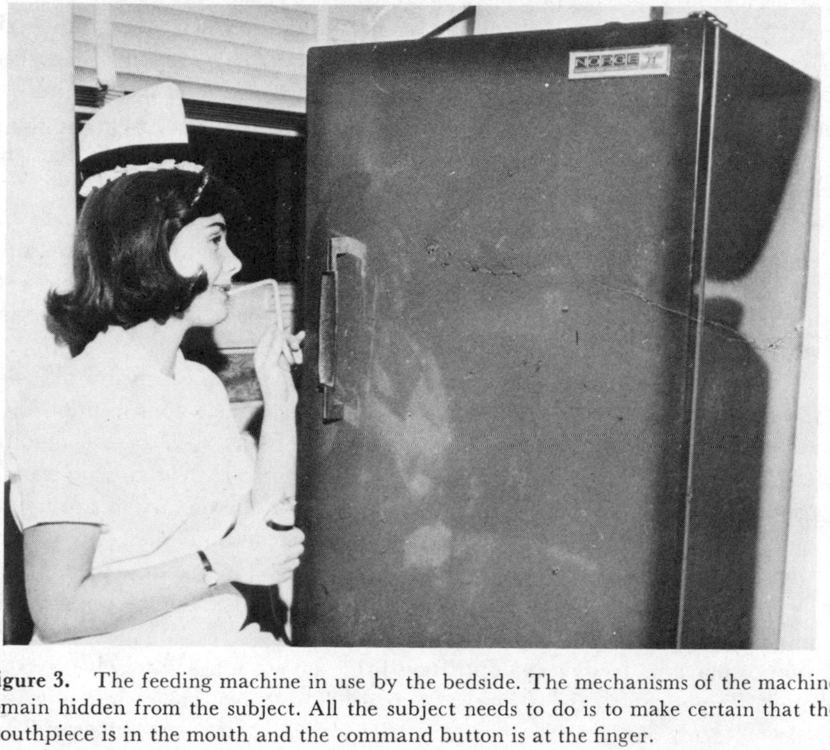

Figure 3. The feeding machine in use by the bedside. The mechanisms of the machine remain hidden from the subject. All the subject needs to do is to make certain that the mouthpiece is in the mouth and the command button is at the finger.

Whenever the subject is engaged in eating the door to the room is closed. The subject is of course confined to the metabolic ward and physical activity is not varied from day to day, as evidenced by activity diaries. During machine feeding the subject realizes fully that the formula is the only source of food. Plain tea, black coffee, and water are allowed as desired.

Certain hypotheses concerning the feeding machine were formulated. Some have been tested; others remain to be substantiated. These are: (1) A normal subject will spontaneously obtain enough food from the machine to maintain body weight over a prolonged period. (2) If body weight is maintained and calorie expenditure virtually constant, a baseline calorie intake and coefficient of variation can be established for a given subject. Such a baseline will make it possible to evaluate and compound the effects of (a) a sustained increase or decrease in energy expenditure; (b) caloric dilution or concentration of the formula diet, or other changes in nutrient composition; (c) pharmacologic agents affecting appetite; (d) changes in external cues, such as dispensing the same formula from a glass rather than from the machine. (3) An abnormal subject (e.g., one with obesity, anorexia nervosa, or prolonged starvation) will respond differently to the feeding machine than a normal lean subject.

Some of these predictions have been answered from the results with the feeding machine (27). Lean healthy adults feeding themselves spontaneously by machine within the confines of the metabolic ward are capable of ingesting sufficient calories to maintain a constant body weight. The button pressing activity is most intense at those times of the day corresponding approximately to the times of breakfast, luncheon, and dinner. Moreover, some food ingestion occurred ("snacks") at midmorning, midafternoon, and late evening. The subjects, of course, remained aware of the time of day, but could not monitor their intake or the composition of the formula diet. There were some daily variations in the calorie intake, but the subjects kept up their food intake by machine without weight loss or weight gain for periods varying from 7 to 51 days.

By contrast, obese subjects feeding themselves spontaneously by machine diminish their food intake drastically (compared to their consumption on a regular hospital diet) to calorie levels that are 10 to 20% of the amount needed to maintain their obese weight. Thus, an obese individual who usually consumes 5000 calories at home (estimated from a dietary history) eats virtually all of the ingredients of a 2800-calorie hospital diet. Thereafter, within the same hospital environment, when changed to machine feeding, the same obese individual drops his calorie intake down to 500 calories without complaining of "hunger." Consequently, he loses weight. When an interim period of machine feeding is stopped and the subject is asked to self-serve the formula (identical to the formula dispensed by machine) by cup, calorie intake goes up significantly to 800 to 1000 calories per day, albeit still far below the level consumed on a self-selected diet. It is evident from these studies that the feeding machine situation offers the obese person a monotonous way of eating. In this way, food-related cues are virtually eliminated and the obese individual settles down to a calorie intake commensurate with his physiologic and nutritional needs. When food-related cues return, food intake increases not in response to physiologic hunger, but in compliance with "external" environmental cues that surround food and food eating situations.

Our group (28) went on to study the effect of covert changes in the nutritive density of a liquid formula diet on food intake in adult lean and obese subjects feeding themselves spontaneously by machine. During periods of alternate caloric dilution and concentration unbeknown to the subject, lean subjects adjust the volume intake of the formula diet and consequently maintain a near constant energy intake and body weight. Physical activity remains virtually unchanged during the alternate periods of change in the caloric density. By contrast, the obese subjects ingested only a small fraction of the calories needed to maintain their weight. Moreover, there is no increase in volume intake in response to formula dilution and no decrease in volume intake after formula concentration. Comparisons of food intake of normal and obese subjects consuming regular foods at home and in the hospital and formula diets dispensed by machine in the hospital are shown in Table 1. These comparisons reveal that lean individuals consume approximately the same amount of calories regardless of the environment or form in which they are presented. By contrast, obese persons consume enormous amounts of calories in their home environment. In the hospital they appear to "settle" for less of regular food. Also in the hospital, when confronted with an eating

Table 1 Food Intake (kilocalories per day) of Adult Lean and Obese Subjects[a]

Subjects	Diet at home (estimated)	Diet in hospital (prescribed)	Self-feeding by machine of formula, 1 cal/ml	Self-feeding by machine of formula, 0.5 kcal/ml Adjustment[b]	Self-feeding by machine of formula, 1.5 kcal/ml Adjustment[b]
Normal	2000	2000	2000	+	+
Obese	4000	2000	500	–	–

[a] The figures are approximate.

[b] Adjustments in response to covert changes in caloric density occur by appropriate change in volume intake.

situation that is devoid of food-related cues, such as the feeding machine, their food intake drops strikingly. When the food cues return, food intake increases, and when such cues become "infinite" in their usual living environment in our society, food intake becomes vastly in excess of their physiologic requirement.

VARIABLES COMPLICATING THE NORMAL EATING PROCESS

There are many variables that influence eating in our daily living. Such variables render the food intake in man difficult to study and often impossible to quantify. However, recognition of some of these variables may have relevance to our food intake behavior.

1. Persons have learned the quantity of a recognizable food that is appropriate in a "normal" meal. Thus, they have been provided with the capability to monitor calorie and nutrient content of a "normal" meal.
2. Most subjects have been taught to "finish" what is placed before them, even if hunger is no longer present.
3. The amount and quality of food consumed may be strongly influenced by learned preferences.
4. Human beings are accustomed to taking food as "'meals" three times a day.
5. There is often an "administrative" delay of variable duration between the time that the person decides that he or she wants food and the time that the food is obtained.
6. Some rich and highly palatable foods may be consumed regularly in the absence of hunger, e.g., desserts, cheeses, coffee or tea with cream and sugar, liqueurs, etc.
7. Usually, food is consumed in a setting in which external cues may be of great importance in determining the amount of food eaten.

Thus, satiety in man living a sedentary life in a developed and industrialized society is subject to modification, overriding, and deletion.

CONCLUSION

The study of hunger and satiety in man is difficult because of the complex nature of human eating behavior. In contrast to lower animals, the process in human beings is an intricate mixture of physiologic, psychologic, cultural, and aesthetic factors. In a society living in an environment such as the United States where food is readily available, people eat not only to satisfy physiologic hunger, but also in response to forces in the environment. When energy expenditure rises, the excess food eaten will be dissipated as energy balance is restored and constancy of body weight is maintained. However, in our society the opportunities for physical activity have diminished markedly. Those who resist the "temptation" to eat more and exercise less emerge as the lean normals as they pass into adulthood. However, a high proportion of our population succumbs to the "temptation" and becomes obese either early or in adult life. Recent studies of food intake in man indicate that there is a need to restructure our food intake behavior by de-emphasizing the forces and pressures in the environment that appear to override our internal physiological needs.

REFERENCES

1. Comstock, G. W. and Stone, R. W. *Arch. Environm. Health* **24**:271 (1972).
2. Chinn, S., Garrow, J. S., and Miall, W. B. In *Energy Balance and Obesity in Man*. North-Holland, London, 1974.
3. Mayer, J. *Nut. Abstr. Rev.* **25**:597; 871 (1955).
4. Mayer, J., Marshall, N. B., Vitale, J. J., Christensen, J. H., Mashayekhi, M. B., and Stare, F. J. *Am. J. Physiol.* **177**:544 (1954).
5. Brozek, J. *Fed. Proc.* **11**:784 (1952).
6. Forbes, G. and Reina, J. C. *Metabolism* **19**:653 (1970).
7. Sims, E. A. H., Goldman, R. F., Gluck, C. M., et al. *Trans. Assoc. Am. Phys.* **81**:531 (1968).
8. Sims, E. A. H., Danforth, E., Jr., Horton, E. S., et al. *Rec. Progr. Horm. Res.* **29**:547 (1973).
9. Cohn, C. and Joseph, D. *Yale J. Biol. Med.* **34**:598 (1962).
10. Van Itallie, T. B. and Campbell, R. G. *J. Am Dietet. Assn.* **61**:385 (1972).
11. Bray, G. A. *Fed. Proc.* **33**:1140 (1974).
12. Bray, G. A. *Metabolism* **24**:99 (1975).
13. Stuart, R. B. and Davis, B. Slim Chance in a Fat World: Behavioral Control of Obesity. Research Press, Champaign, Ill., 1972.
14. Jordan, H. A. and Levitz, L. S. *Obesity Bariatric Med.* **4**:58 (1975).
15. Stunkard, A. J. and Koch, C. *Arch. Gen Psychiat.* **11**:74 (1964).
16. Schachter, S., Goldman, R., and Gordon, A. *J. Person. Soc. Psychol.* **10**:91 (1968).
17. Schachter, S. *Science* **161**:751 (1968).
18. Nisbett, R. E. *Science* **159**:1254 (1968).
19. Ross, L. D. Ph.D. dissertation, Columbia University, 1970.
20. Deck, E. In *Emotion, Obesity, and Crime*, S. Schachter, Ed., Academic, New York, 1971, p. 103.
21. Schachter, S. *Am. Psychologist* **26**:129 (1971).

22. Schachter, S. and Rodin, J. *Obese Humans and Rats*. Erlbaum-Halsted, Washington, D.C., 1974.
23. Skinner, B. F. *Behavior of Organisms*. Appleton, New York, 1938.
24. Anliker, J. and Mayer, J. *J. Appl. Physiol.* **8**:667 (1956).
25. Teitelbaum, P. *J. Comp. Physiol.* **48**:156 (1955).
26. Hashim, S. A. and Van Itallie, T. B. *Fed Proc.* 23 (part 1, No. 1):**82** (1964).
27. Hashim, S. A. and Van Itallie, T. B. *Ann. N.Y. Acad. Sci.* **131**:654 (1965).
28. Campbell, R. G., Mashim, S. A., and Van Itallie, T. B. *New Eng. J. Med.* **285**: 1402 (1972).

10

Adipose Tissue Cellularity and its Relationship to the Development of Obesity in Females

M. R. C. GREENWOOD, Ph.D.

Institute of Human Nutrition, College of Physicians and Surgeons, Columbia University, New York, New York

and

PATRICIA R. JOHNSON, Ph.D.

Department of Biology, Vassar College, Poughkeepsie, New York

The American woman is concerned about obesity. In her role as wife and homemaker, she bears responsibility not only for her own health and well-being, but for that of her family as well. In our multimedia society, she is continually bombarded with information concerning not only how to feed her family in a healthful way, but also about the need to remain slim and beautiful herself. She may avail herself of any of the more than 17,000 weight reduction methods that have been published to date. She, perhaps more than the average American male, is made increasingly aware that obesity is one of the nation's major public health problems, and that while it is not a problem of women exclusively, it does have a higher incidence in women than in men.

According to a recent report (1), the prevalence of obesity among American men in each decade from age 35 to 74 was approximately 15%, while in women it was 20% in the 35 to 44 age group, but had reached 30% by

Some of the research reported herein was supported in part by NIH grants HD–8965, HD–02761 and by grants from the Research Corporation and the Nutrition Foundation.

55 years of age. In addition to this data from the United States, studies that confirm these trends have been reported from other countries as well. In a Czechoslovakian community that was assessed for the prevalence of obesity in 1956 and reexamined in 1971, Oscanova (2) reported that the incidence of obesity in men in all age groups from 20 to 50 had at least doubled by 1971 compared to 1956. In women, the incidence of obesity in the younger (20 to 30) age groups did not change over the period studied, while in the 35 years of age or older groups, the prevalence increased. In women who were 50 or older, the figures reached 60%. Thus, despite the evidence of concern over the problems of increased body weight, increasingly more women who live in today's affluent societies are apparently fighting a losing battle.

Woman's concern with body size and weight and its relationship to aesthetic standards has a long tradition. Aesthetic standards, however, change over time, and thus it is necessary to note that what was considered a normal and attractive weight for women during certain periods of history would by today's slim standards be considered obese. Many examples of feminine pulchritude depicted in early Greek and Roman sculpture, and certainly many of those in the Rubens masterpieces would be considered candidates for the latest method of weight reduction in today's society. Thus, while the modern woman may well be more aware of body weight ranges that are consistent with optimum health standards than her forebears, she finds herself constantly bombarded with marketing messages that encourage an aesthetic standard inconsistent with the realities of an affluent society.

The statistics on treatment leave no doubt that there are no "cures" for obesity. While almost any method of weight reduction will produce some degree of weight loss in the motivated obese individual, maintenance of the reduced body weight rarely occurs (in something less than 10% of all reported studies) (3, 4). One must conclude that the only way to reduce the prevalence of obesity is to prevent its occurrence. What is understood about the etiology of obesity? Are there specific times at which intervention might lead to prevention?

Obesity occurs as an abnormality of caloric balance reflected in the increased deposition of lipid in adipose tissue. It is generally accepted that the amount of calories stored in adipose tissue is the result of calories ingested minus the calories utilized for body maintenance and activity. A defect in regulation of the homeostatic balance between "calories in, calories out, and calories stored," leads to physiologically inappropriate leanness or fatness.

Numerous factors have been implicated in the regulation of caloric intake and body weight, and a dysfunction of any, or a combination of them, can lead to the production and maintenance of the obese condition. The factors which are known to be involved in the normal regulation of body weight and which are altered in the obese, range from cognitive factors related to the mode of food intake (5, 6, 7), to neurohormonal factors that have been implicated in short-term (8, 9, 10, 11), or long-term (12) regulation of food intake, to alterations in hypothalamic function (13, 14), to changes in hormonal status (15), to the effects of early nutritional status (16, 17), to genetic endowment (18), to decreased activity (19, 20), and to differences in adipose tissue morphology (21, 22, 23, 24). Our own studies have focused on the role of adipose tissue morphology and how it develops and changes in the obese.

ADIPOSE TISSUE CELLULARITY IN HUMANS

Types of Obesity

In 1968 Hirsch and his colleagues developed a rapid technique for determining the number and size of fat cells in humans and made the exciting discovery that at least some obese humans had many more fat cells than normal weight humans (25). After an extensive examination of fat cellularity in humans, they were able to suggest that fat cell number and size were important determinants of the type of obesity present in an individual. Their data suggested that at least two types of obesity could be distinguished on the basis of adipose tissue morphology: (a) a hyperplastic-hypertrophic form and (b) a hypertrophic form. In the population used for these studies, those individuals with a history of very early onset of obesity were primarily of the hyperplastic-hypertrophic type, whereas individuals who reported an onset of obesity later in life were primarily of the hypertrophic variety. The currently available cellularity data on obese individuals are sparse enough that they do not rule out still other morphological classifications of the obese condition. The concept that early onset obesity is often accompanied by hyperplasia is greatly strengthened by the data of Brook and co-workers (26) in England, and Bjorntorp and co-workers in Sweden (27), who have reported similar results. Figure 1 shows that the fat cell number of normal weight adult women and men is similar and is between 20 and 40 billion cells. American women and men have similar values for the normal range (26). However, among the obese individuals studied by Brook (26), there are two types of obese men and women. Those individuals in whom the obesity occurred as early as one year of age were the individuals who showed increased numbers of fat cells as adults, while those who became obese as adults showed primarily fat cell enlargement with little or no change in fat cell number.

Knittle and associates have demonstrated that different patterns of fat cellularity development are apparent in obese and nonobese children (28). Figure 2 shows the data collected on nonobese children from 2 to 18 years of age. In the normal, nonobese child fat cell numbers in the adult range are not reached until 8 to 12 years of age (29). Knittle has suggested that the attain-

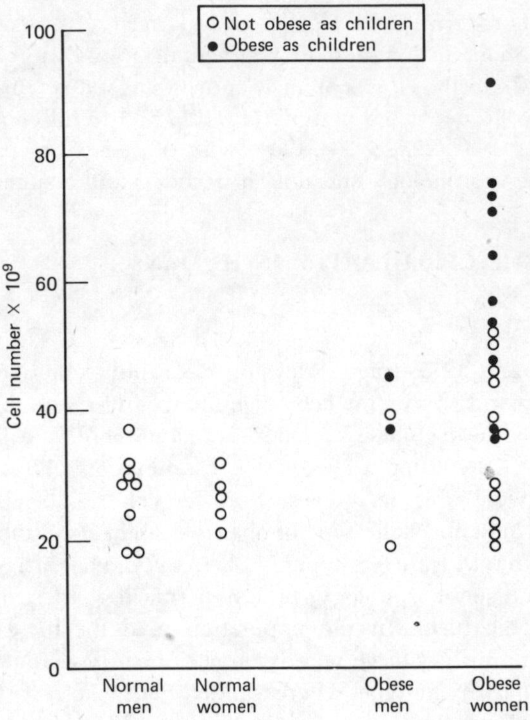

Figure 1. Total number of adipose cells in adults. From Brook and co-workers, *British Medical Journal*, 2:25 (1972).

ment of adult values comes about as a result of two critical periods of cellular proliferation: one from birth to 2 years of age and another preceding puberty (29). In the obese child, this pattern may be fundamentally different (Fig. 3). Obese children show increments in fat cell number throughout the period studied and seem to increase fat cell number throughout childhood and early adolescence rather than only during two critical periods (Fig. 3). Furthermore, when studied longitudinally, individual obese children show marked increments in fat cell number over a two-year period, while nonobese children studied over the same ages show no change in fat cell number (29). The causes for the marked adipocyte hyperplasia in obese children are currently unknown, but both early nutrition (16) and genetic endowment (18) have been implicated.

Normal Weight Adult Women

Krotkiewski and co-workers (30) reported a study of 31 randomly selected

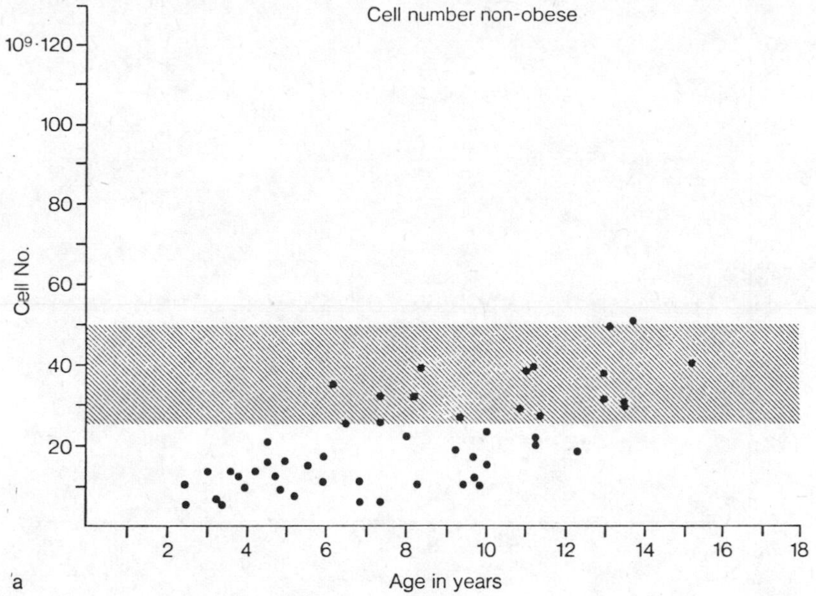

Figure 2. Adipose cell number as a function of age in nonobese children. The hatched area represents normal nonobese adult range. From Knittle, J. L., *Triangle* (*Sandoz Journal of Medical Science*), **13**(2):60 (1974).

Swedish women 52 years of age, and 13 young women with a mean age of 22. All of the women were normal weight. As a group the 52-year-old women, while of normal body weight, were significantly fatter. This change in body composition was the result of increased body fat (BF) and decreased body cell mass (BCM) and is consistent with findings from many other laboratories. Table 1 shows that the increased fat in 52-year-old normal weight women is a result of larger than normal fat cells, not elevated fat cell number. Perhaps of even more interest is the finding that the younger women, although of normal weight, had more fat cells than the older women. This finding remains consistent when the young and older women are matched for height, body weight, or for body fat. Although not extremely hyperplastic as obese children appear to be, these young women are consistently in the upper ranges or slightly above normal range for adult fat cell numbers. The Swedish investigators suggest the possibility that the younger group of women may have more fat cells as a result of better nutrition, or perhaps overnutrition, early in life (30). These results have focused interest once again on the factors that affect the early development of adipose tissue.

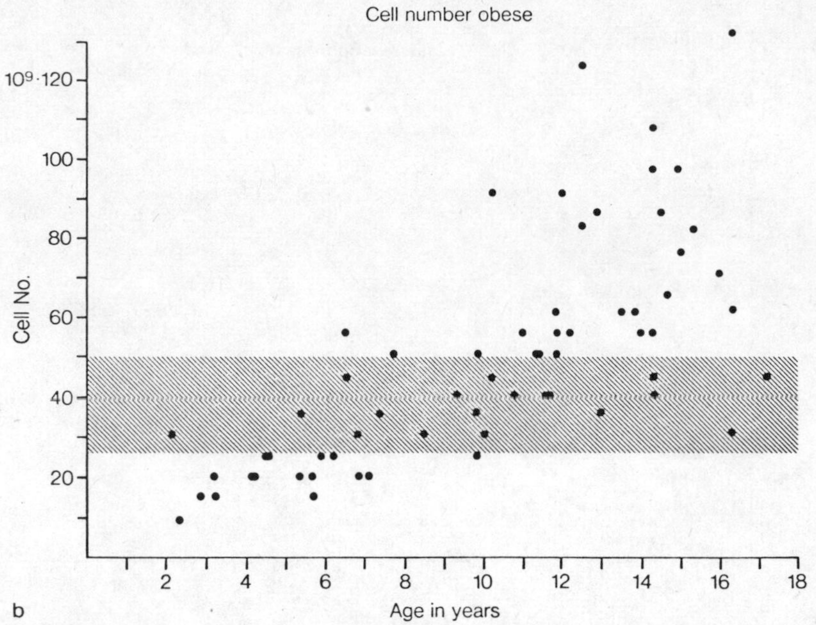

Figure 3. Adipose cell number as a function of age in obese children. The hatched area represents normal nonobese adult range. From Knittle, J. L., *Triangle* (*Sandoz Journal of Medical Science*), **13**(2):60 (1974).

Table 1 Adipose Tissue Cellularity in Normal Weight Young and Middle-Aged Women[a]

	n	Size (μg/lipid)	Fat Cell Number ($\times 10^9$)
Young	9	0.32 ± 0.02	36.0 ± 3.5
Middle-aged	9	0.56 ± 0.04	27.6 ± 3.0
(height matched)			
p		< .001	< .05
Young	13	0.31 ± 0.02	41.4 ± 5.3
Middle-aged	13	0.51 ± 0.03	26.4 ± 1.6
(body weight matched)			
p		< .001	< .01
Young	13	0.31 ± 0.02	41.4 ± 5.4
Middle-aged	13	0.53 ± 0.02	23.0 ± 1.8
(body fat matched)			
p		< .001	< .01

[a] Data from (30).

ADIPOSE TISSUE CELLULARITY IN OBESE FEMALE RATS

In our attempts to explore animal models useful in studying the development of obesity, we have utilized female Zucker rats. This strain of rat described by Zucker and Zucker in 1961 carries a recessive gene for obesity (fa), but the obese rats (fa/fa) do not breed. Therefore, it is necessary to breed heterozygous lean rats (Fa/fa) to produce the homozygous recessive genotype. In litters from such matings (Fa/fa x Fa/fa), obese pups (fa/fa) occur 25% of the time while the remaining pups are lean, either heterozygous or homozygous (Fa/fa and Fa/Fa). The growth and development of adipose tissue cellularity in the male of this strain has been described by Johnson and co-workers (31, 32). Recently, in collaboration with Drs. Stern, Batchelor, and Hirsch (33), we have described the sequential development of adipocyte hyperplasia as well as the accompanying hyperinsulinemia and insulin resistance in the female obese Zucker rat.

Female Zucker obese rats are significantly heavier than their nonobese litter mates as early as 3 weeks of age and by 9 weeks of age there is a clear separation of lean and obese body weights (Table 2). This difference in body weight is due to increasing adiposity. The obese rat is fatter at all ages

Table 2 Body Composition in Female Zucker Rats

	Lean			Obese		
Age (wks)	Body Weight (n) (g)	Total Fat (g)	Carcass Weight (g)	Body Weight (n) (g)	Total Fat (g)	Carcass Weight (g)
5	112.0	2.264	45.6	150.2	22.669	43.6
	(n = 6)	±0.403	±1.8	(n = 6)	±1.302	±1.8
8	158.7	5.412	69.9	219.7	51.526	40.8
	(n = 3)	±0.670	±2.0	(n = 3)	±1.224	±3.9
9	192.7	5.835	85.2	309.3	68.989	89.2
	(n = 6)	±0.711	±3.0	(n = 6)	±3.047	±2.0
14	221.8	9.120	109.5	460.3	138.065	121.9
	(n = 6)	±1.380	±2.1	(n = 4)	±10.337	±2.4
24	266.5	18.723	127.9	578.2	208.634	147.3
	(n = 6)	±2.154	±2.4	(n = 5)	±12.631	±6.0
36	304.7	22.122	147.5	613.8	240.674	156.2
	(n = 6)	±2.616	±6.1	(n = 5)	±13.748	±9.6
52	279.7	16.375	134.0	730.0	298.982	180.2
	(n = 6)	±2.622	±4.2	(n = 2)	±35.624	±3.3

sampled, while carcass weight of obese females does not differ from lean females except at one year where only two fatty rats were examined (Table 2). These findings are in accord with those presented by Bell and Stern (34) who showed that body fat was elevated in the obese male rat as early as 13 days of age.

The growth and development of the adipose tissue was investigated by examining three dissectible sites—the gonadal, or parametrial fat pad, the retroperitoneal fat pad, and the dorsal scapular subcutaneous fat pad. Total animal fat cellularity was calculated from total dissectible fat and three depots as previously described (31).

The data for the cellularity determinations in the three sites are shown in Table 3. As is typical of most rat strains, the lean female rat (Fa/–) of the Zucker strain shows a gradual increase in pad weight until 18 to 20 weeks of age, after which the pad weight remains essentially constant. In the lean female, as in the lean male (31), this growth is accompanied by increases in cell number measured by electronic counting of osmium-fixed fat cells until 16 to 20 weeks of age, after which adult fat cell number does not change. Fat cell size also shows steady increments until 14 weeks of age, decreasing slightly and leveling off at the older ages.

The pattern is very different in the obese rat (Table 3). The fat pad continues to increase in weight beyond 20 weeks of age. This change in weight is accompanied by marked increases in fat cell number and fat cell size. This strikingly different pattern is clearly obvious in all three sites.

When the data are calculated as average cell size and total fat cellularity, it is clear that the pattern of development of cell size and number in the obese female is fundamentally different from that of the lean female (Table 4). We have noted a peak cell size at 14 weeks of age and have further suggested that it is coincident with a sharp increase in the pattern of increasing fat cell number. These data led us to speculate that this peak cell size might in some way act as a stimulus to further fat cell proliferation (33, 35) in the obese. Our most recent investigations have been toward elucidating this point.

One of the serious limitations of the method utilizing electronic counting of osmium-fixed fat cells, as well as of many histometric techniques, is that these techniques are only useful in detecting fat cells that contain a critical level of lipid. Therefore, such methods cannot detect "preadipocytes," i.e., cells that will become filled with lipid. Such methods tell us not when fat cells are made, but rather, when they fill with lipid. Some of this difficulty of interpretation was alleviated by utilizing a method to study H^3-thymidine incorporation into DNA of precursor fat cells (36). These thymidine incorporation studies in normal lean Sprague-Dawley male rats demonstrated (Figs. 4 and 5) that few, if any, new fat cells are made after the fourth or fifth postnatal week. Since the H^3-thymidine incorporation studies are very

Table 3 Adipose Tissue Cellularity from Three Sites in Lean and Obese Females

		Subcutaneous			Gonadal			Retroperitoneal		
Weeks	(n)	Wet Wt.	Cell Size	Cell No. $\times 10^6$	Wet Wt.	Cell Size	Cell No. $\times 10^6$	Wet Wt.	Cell Size	Cell 10×10^6
					Lean					
5	(6)	512.6	0.0484	3.717	79.2	0.0320	1.276	46.7	0.0541	0.615
		±77.9	±0.0122	±0.162	±13.8	±0.0045	±0.242	±8.5	±0.0195	±0.134
8	(3)	794.9	0.0596	5.916	408.5	0.0909	3.391	199.9	0.0885	1.551
		±85.3	±0.0000	0.363	±66.1	±0.0063	±0.329	±14.1	±0.0063	±0.218
9	(6)	1168.9	0.0699	7.639	426.8	0.1116	2.815	239.3	0.1165	—
		±109.4	±0.0095	±1.013	±74.2	±0.0155	±0.297	±31.7	±0.0207	
14	(6)	1920.9	0.0919	10.025	986.1	0.2460	3.535	395.9	0.2380	1.469
		±242.9	±0.0161	±0.641	±134.0	±0.0487	±0.450	±60.6	±0.0545	±0.175
24	(6)	3197.9	0.1829	9.502	2353.3	0.4833	4.082	1055.3	0.4394	1.919
		±359.1	±0.0253	±0.865	±377.0	±0.0574	±0.206	±152.7	±0.0391	±0.129
36	(6)	4020.2	0.2031	10.849	2992.7	0.5124	4.943	1187.4	0.4637	2.154
		519.4	0.0298	1.116	412.2	0.0592	0.310	129.0	0.0823	0.329
52	(6)	2472.9	0.1449	9.058	2344.0	0.3724	5.191	1011.3	0.3688	2.170
		±323.0	±0.0145	±0.852	±496.0	±0.0487	±0.606	±166.2	±0.0356	±0.321
					Obese					
5	(6)	4108.3	0.6359	5.066	1232.3	0.4681	2.291	508.8	0.5062	0.826
		±261.9	±0.0259	±0.234	±111.6	±0.0510	±0.195	±48.3	±0.0293	±0.073
8	(3)	10631.5	1.0530	8.214	4375.7	1.0111	3.737	1854.7	0.8399	1.881
		±1200.4	±0.0974	±1.861	±312.3	±0.0775	±0.388	±137.8	±0.1222	±0.158
9	(6)	13428.3	1.1212	9.296	6413.8	1.3794	4.267	3012.2	1.1726	2.188
		±825.2	±0.0936	±0.786	±146.3	±0.1894	±0.450	±180.1	±0.0635	±0.210
14	(4)	30423.2	1.7721	14.058	12377.4	2.4785	4.626	6199.6	1.8628	2.973
		±3841.0	±0.0955	±1.397	±395.9	±0.2261	±0.477	±504.4	±0.0995	±0.352
24	(5)	51396.0	1.2409	33.013	12985.7	1.6981	6.916	16171.5	1.5019	9.742
		±728.0	±0.0752	±7.994		±0.1833	±0.671	±137.4	±0.0197	±1.275
36	(5)	70881.8	1.3429	42.593	15127.7	1.7115	7.979	19826.4	1.4498	12.116
		3120.4	0.1760	±7.408	±739.9	±0.1378	±0.637	±970.5	±0.0628	±0.965
52	(2)	90124.6	1.3624	55.623	151021.6	1.8031	8.010	24613.2	1.4361	16.121
		±4011.7	±0.1831	±5.602	±803.7	±0.1461	±0.236	±987.4	±0.0521	±0.821

Table 4 Total Adipose Tissue Cellularity in Lean and Obese Female Zucker Rats

	Lean			Obese		
Age (wk)	(n)	Cell Number × 10^6	Cell size μg lipid	n	Cell Number × 10^6	Cell size μg lipid
5	6	17.583 ±0.703	0.0461 ±0.0105	6	30.012 ±1.611	0.6013 ±0.0255
8	3	41.480 ±5.421	0.0668 ±0.0000	3	40.486 ±3.744	1.0241 ±0.0954
9	6	37.407 ±3.407	0.0799 ±0.0114	6	48.413 ±2.813	1.1595 ±0.0941
14	6	44.671 ±1.634	0.1141 ±0.0221	4	60.996 ±3.861	1.8888 ±0.1173
24	6	47.585 ±3.406	0.2558 ±0.0868	5	126.849 ±20.220	1.3555 ±0.0974
36	6	51.014 ±3.418	0.2852 ±0.0404	5	141.422 ±16.035	1.3834 ±0.1452
52	6	50.115 ±4.881	0.2110 ±0.0230	2	174.457 ±3.456	1.3700 ±0.1416

tedious and can never be applied to humans, attempts have been made to develop enzymatic methods that do not require radioisotope administration to monitor these stages of growth (37, 38).

Cleary and associates have reported that thymidine kinase, one of the enzymes that provides precursors for DNA synthesis, is an accurate monitor of the rate of preadipocyte division and correlates well with experiments on thymidine incorporation into DNA in normal lean rats (37). Furthermore, it was demonstrated that the activity of this enzyme is elevated in male obese Zucker rats, compared to age-matched lean rats (37). The obese female Zucker rat also shows a significant elevation in thymidine kinase activity in adipose tissue at 14 weeks of age over that level seen in lean female rats, but at 26 weeks of age the elevated level is no longer measurable (33).

Another demonstration that new cells may be being added in the female at this age is suggested by examining the distribution of cell diameters in obese and lean rats (Fig. 6). As expected, obese females have larger fat cells than lean rats. The fat cell diameter is in agreement with the average fat cell size calculated by our usual methods. However, the obese rat appears to have a bimodal distribution of fat cells at 15½ weeks of age, which is not seen in the

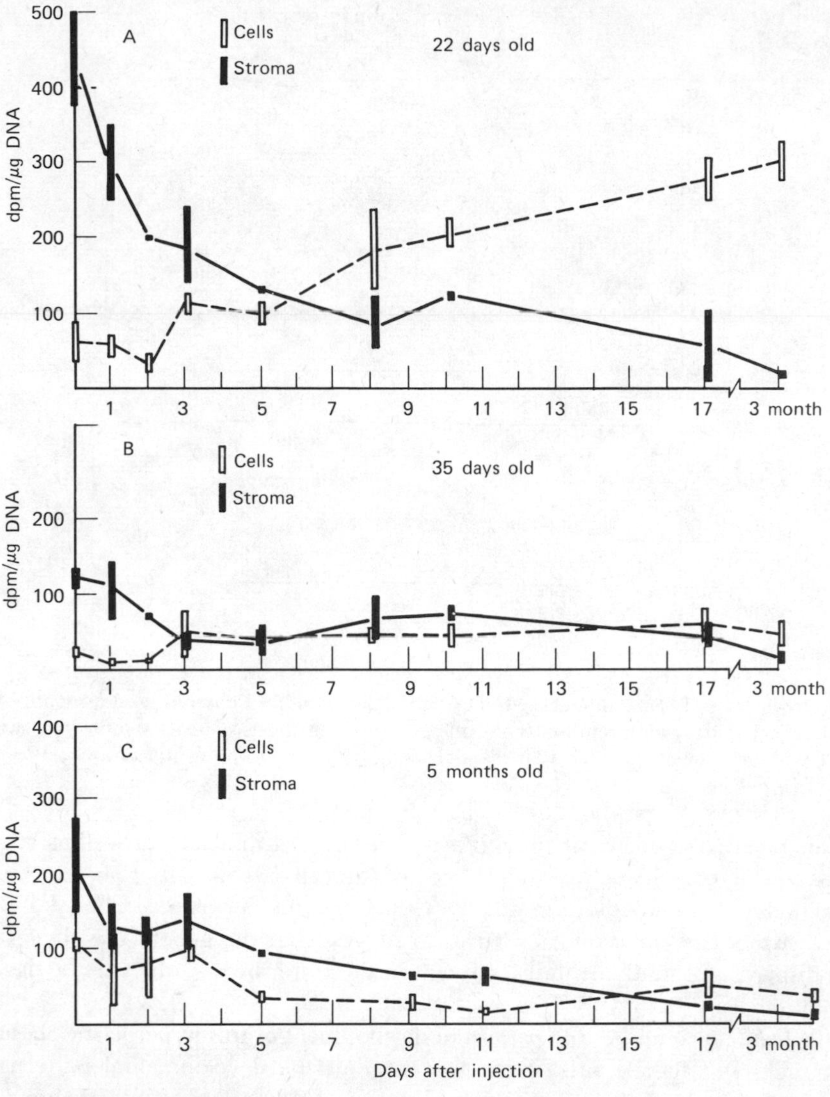

Figure 4. In vivo injection H^3-thymidine; specific activity of adipocyte and stromal fractions. Open bars and dotted lines represent the specific activity determined at various times postinjection in the isolated adipocyte fraction. Closed bars and solid lines represent the specific activity determined in the stromal-vascular fraction. Bars represent the ranges of the two pools sampled at each time point. From Greenwood, M. R. C. and Hirsch, J. *Journal of Lipid Research*, **15**:474 (1974).

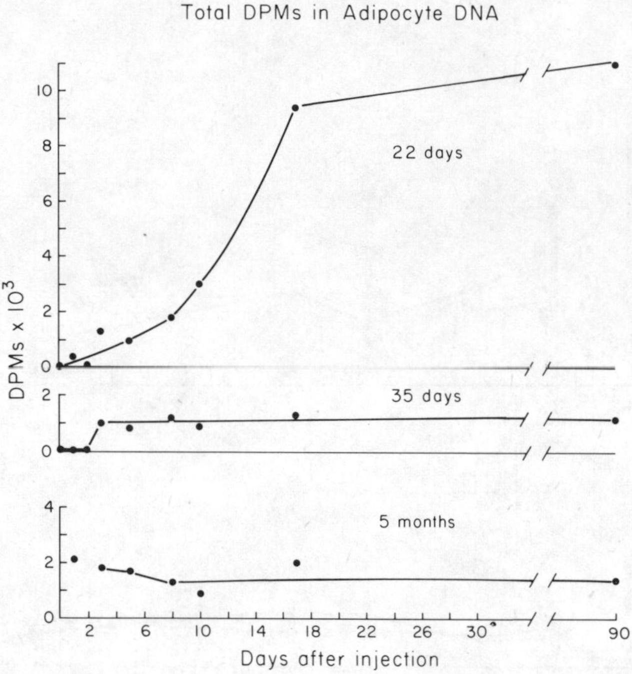

Figure 5. Total dpms in adipocyte DNA for 22-day-old, 35-day-old, and 5-month-old rats. Each data point represents the mean value for the two pools sampled at each time. From Greenwood, M. R. C. and Hirsch, J. *Journal of Lipid Research*, **15:**474 (1974).

lean rat. In the obese rat there is a population of small cells as well as large cells. The coincidence of this bimodal fat cell size distribution, elevated thymidine kinase activity in adipose tissue, and the occurrence of a peak fat cell size in the obese rat, has led us to suggest that the genetically obese rat is displaying a fundamentally different pattern of growth in its adipose tissue than the lean rat (35).

When one compares the pattern of development of this hyperplastic obesity in male and female rats, it is apparent that the developmental pattern is basically similar between the sexes with a few subtle differences. There are usual sex differences with respect to body weight increments. The lean female rat attains adult body weight early, while the male continues to grow. Nonetheless, the pattern of cellular growth in adipose tissue is similar between the sexes.

A comparison of the developing pattern of fat cellularity in the retroperitoneal fat pad of obese and lean male and female rats is shown in Table 5.

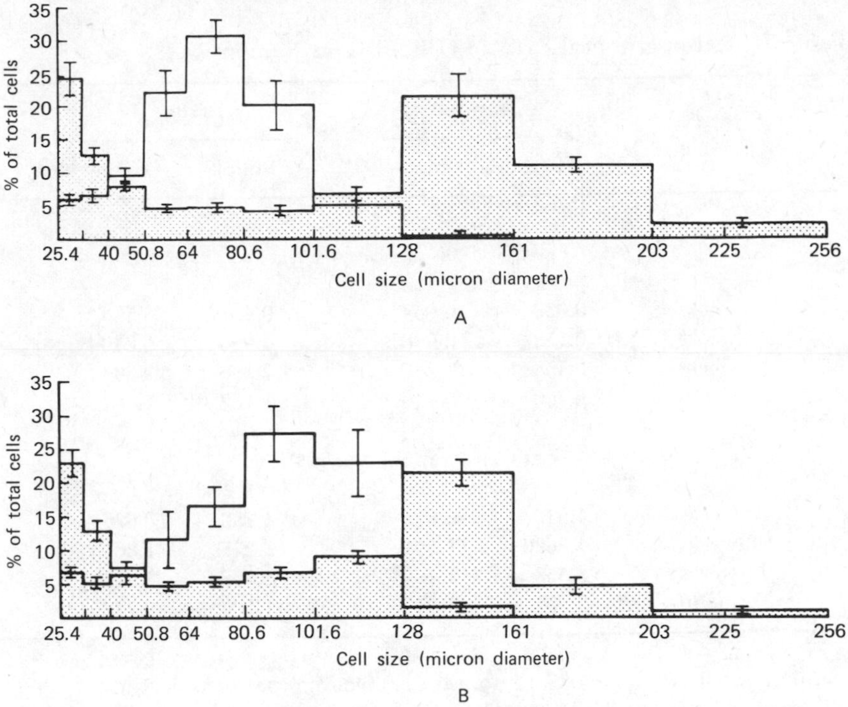

Figure 6. Distribution of adipocyte diameters in obese and lean 15-week-old Zucker rats. (A) Distribution of cell diameters in the subcutaneous depot. (B) Distribution of cell diameters in the retroperitoneal depot.

In both sexes, fat cell size increases with age. Fat cell number increases in the lean rats of both sexes until 14 weeks of age. In the obese rats of both sexes, fat cell number continues to increase until at least 6 months of age. Lean male rats have larger fat cells at all ages than females, but female obese rats have larger fat cells at all ages than obese male rats. In general, there are no fundamental differences in fat cellularity between the sexes in either lean or obese. The major differences in cellularity are related to genotype. In both male and female genetically obese rats there appears to be a fundamentally different pattern of control for fat cell proliferation compared to lean rats.

One obvious question to be derived from these findings is, "Can they be extrapolated to the human condition?" Such a question is difficult to answer because it is still not known whether obesity may be an inherited trait in women and men. Statistically, one has an increasing chance of becoming obese if one has an obese or two obese parents (18, 39). What is not yet clear is whether this statistic may be due to inherited endowment, to early over-

Table 5 Retroperitoneal Fat Pad Cell Size and Number

Age	Fa/–		fa/fa	
	Male	Female	Male	Female
	Fat Cell Size (μg Lipid/Cell)			
5 weeks	0.038	0.054	0.451	0.506
8 weeks	0.153	0.098	0.990	0.840
14 weeks	0.458	0.258	1.436	1.863
6 months	0.700	0.440	1.182	1.502
	Fat Cell Number ($\times 10^6$)			
5 weeks	1.613	0.615	1.252	0.826
8 weeks	1.8636	1.551	2.245	1.881
14 weeks	3.558	1.469	4.606	2.973
6 months	2.981	1.919	11.186	9.742

feeding, or to early exposure to family feeding patterns leading to over-ingestion. The Swedish study (30) suggests that early overnutrition in humans may be a potential stimulus for extra fat cell proliferation. In lean rats, over-nutrition can increase fat cell number, although not to the degree seen in genetically obese rats (32). Furthermore, in the presence of the obese gene, early overnutrition has the even more devastating effect of further increasing fat cell number (32).

Although there is currently some discussion among investigators (40) about the timing of fat cell proliferation in normal and obese humans, investigators agree that once fat cells are acquired, they are not lost through dieting. There is also considerable agreement that the longstanding juvenile onset and hyperplastic forms of obesity are the most refractory to treatment. It is also known that most of the metabolic and hormonal changes that accompany the obese state are reversible with weight loss. As fat cell size approaches normal, the usual cellular metabolic and hormonal responsiveness of adipocytes is restored. When an excess number of fat cells is present, in order for the hyperplastic individual to become equivalently thin compared to a non-hyperplastic individual, he or she must reduce the cells to smaller than normal size. Thus, one possible physiological complication of dieting in the case of hyperplastic obesity is that smaller than normal fat cells are produced and they may overrespond to hormonal or substrate signals and erroneously stimulate ingestion to begin the re-eating cycle so commonly seen in obese individuals. Before we can understand with any real sophistication how the number and size of fat cells influence the regulation of food intake, much more work is needed in several disciplines. An understanding of the mechanisms of successful weight loss and better comprehension of the physiological and morphological changes accompanying dieting are necessary in order to produce successful treatments and preventive measures in both women and men.

ACKNOWLEDGMENT

The authors wish to thank M. P. Cleary for performing the thymidine kinase assay and R. Gruen and S. Blanchett-Hirst for doing the adipocyte distribution procedures for us. Since much of the data collected on the female Zucker rat was collected in the laboratory of Dr. Jules Hirsch and with the collaboration of Dr. Judith Stern, we are especially indebted to them.

REFERENCES

1. Heald, F. P. The natural history of obesity. *Adv. Psychosom. Med.* **7**:102 (1972).
2. Oscanova, K. Trends of dietary intake and prevalence of obesity in Czechoslovakia. Recent Advances in Obesity Research: 1, *Proceeding of the 1st International Congress on Obesity*. Ed., Howard Newman, Publ. Ltd. (1975).
3. Stunkard, A. J. and McLaren-Hume, M. The results of treatment for obesity. A review of the literature and report of a Series. *Arch. Intern. Med.* **130**:79 (1959).
4. Stunkard, A. J., Levin, and Fox, S. The management of obesity: Patient self-help and medical treatment. *Arch. Intern. Med.* **125**:1067 (1970).
5. Schachter, S. and Rodin, J. *Obese Humans and Rats*. Lawrence Erlbaum, Potomac, Md., 1974.
6. Le Magnen, J. Regulation of Food Intake. *Adv. Psychosom. Med.* **7**:73 (1972).
7. Grinker, J., Price, J., and Greenwood, M. R. C. Studies of Taste in Childhood Obesity. In *Hunger: Basic Mechanisms and Clinical Implication*. D. Novin, W. Wyrwicka, and G. Bray, Eds., Raven, New York, 1976, pp. 441–57.
8. Gibbs, J., Young, R. C., and Smith, G. P. Cholecystokinin decreases food intake in rats. *J. Comp. Physiol. Psychol.* **84**:488 (1973).
9. Hervey, G. R. Regulation of energy balance. *Nature* **222**:629 (1969).
10. Davis, J. D., Campbell, C. S., Gallagher, R. J., and Zurakou, M. A. Disappearance of a humoral satiety factor during food deprivation. *J. Comp Physiol. Psychol.* **75**:476 (1972).
11. Mayer, J. Regulation of energy intake and the body weight. The glucostatic theory and the lipostatic hypothesis. *Ann. N.Y. Acad. Sci.* **63**:15 (1955).

12. Kennedy, G. C. The role of depot fat in the hypothalamic control of food intake in the rat. *Proc. Roy. Soc.* (Series B). **140**:578 (1953).

13. Bray, G. A. and York, D. A. Studies on food intake in genetically obese rats. *Am. J. Physiol.* **223**:176 (1972).

14. Anand, B. K. and Brobeck, J. R. Hypothalamic control of food intake in rats and cats. *Yale J. Biol. Med.* **24**:123 (1951).

15. Flatt, J. P. Role of the increased adipose tissue mass in the apparent insulin insensitivity of obesity. *Am. J. Clin. Nutr.* **25**:1189 (1972).

16. Knittle, J. L. and Hirsch, J. Effect of early nutrition on the development of rat epididymal fat pads: cellularity and metabolism. *J. Clin. Invest.* **47**:2091 (1968).

17. Hirsch, J. and Han, P. W. Cellularity of rat adipose tissue: effects of growth, starvation and obesity. *J. Lipid Res.* **10**:77 (1969).

18. Mayer, J. Genetic factors in human obesity. *Ann. N.Y. Acad. Sci.* **131**:412 (1965).

19. Mayer, J. *Overweight; Causes, Cost and Control.* Prentice-Hall, Englewood Cliffs, N. J., 1968.

20. Stern, J. S. and Johnson, P. R. Spontaneous activity in the Zucker obese rat (fa fa). *Fed. Proc.* **33**:677 (1974).

21. Johnson, P. R. and Hirsch, J. Cellularity of adipose depots in six strains of genetically obese mice. *J. Lipid Res.* **13**:2 (1972).

22. Helleman, B. and Hellerstrom, C. Cell renewal in the white and brown fat of the rat. *Acta Path. Microbiol. Scand.* **51**:347 (1961).

23. DiGiralomo, M., Thorman, L., and Cullen J. Observations on adipose tissue cellularity and development in rats and rabbits fed *ad lib.* In *Regulation of the Adipose Mass.* J. Vague and J. Bayer, Eds., Excerpta Medica, Amsterdam, 1973.

24. Lemmonier, D. Effect of age, sex and site on the cellularity of adipose tissue in mice and rats rendered obese by a high fat diet. *J. Clin. Invest.* **51**:2907 (1972).

26. Brook, C. Evidence for a sensitive period in adipose cell replication in man *Lancet*, 624 (1972).

27. Bjortorp, P. Disturbances in the regulation of food intake *Adv. Psychosom. Med.* **7**:116 (1972).

28. Knittle, J. L. Obesity in Childhood: a problem in adipose tissue cellular development. *J. Pediatrics* **81**:1048 (1972).

29. Knittle, J. L. In *Nutrient Requirements in Adolescence.* J. I. McKigney and H. Munroe, Eds., MIT Press, Cambridge, Mass., 1976, pp. 75–8.

30. Krotkiewski, M., Sjostrom, L., Bjorntorp. P., and Smith, U. Regional Adipose Tissue Cellularity in relation to metabolism in young and middle-aged women. *Metabolism* **24**:703 (1975).

31. Johnson, P. R., Zucker, L. M., Cruce, J. A. F., and Hirsch, J. Cellularity of adipose depots in the genetically obese Zucker rat. *J. Lipid Res.* **12**:706 (1971).

32. Johnson, P. R., Stern, J. S., Greenwood, M. R. C., Zucker, L. M., and Hirsch, J. Effects of early nutrition on adipose cellularity and pancreatic insulin release in the Zucker rat. *J. Nutr.* **103**:738 (1973).

33. Johnson, P. R., Stern, J. S., Greenwood, M. R. C., Batchelor, B. R., and Hirsch, J. Adipose tissue hyperplasia, hyperinsulinemia and insulin resistance in Zucker obese female rats—a developmental study. Submitted for publication.

34. Bell, G. E. and Stern, J. S. Development of obesity and hyperinsulinemia in the Zucker obese rat (fa fa). *Fed. Proc.* **35**:657 (1976).

35. Johnson, P. R., Stern, J., Gruen, R., Blanchett-Hirst, S., and Greenwood, M. R. C. Development of adipose depot cellularity, plasma insulin, pancreatic insulin release and insulin resistance in the Zucker obese female rat. *Fed. Proc.* **35**:657 1976.

37. Cleary, M. P., Greenwood, M. R. C., and Brasel, J. A. Thymidine kinase as a measure of adipocyte proliferation in normal and obese rats. *Fed. Proc.* **34**:908 (1975).

38. Cleary, M. P., Klein, B. E., Greenwood, M. R. C., and Brasel, J. A. Proliferative enzymes in adipose tissue of normal and obese rats. *Fed. Proc.* **35**:502 (1976).

39. Garn, S. M. and Clark, D. C. Trends in fatness and the origins of obesity. *Pediatrics* **57**:443 (1976).

40. Widdowson, E. and Shaw, W. T. Letters to the editor, *Lancet* **2**:905 (1973).

11

Weight Control Programs

JUDITH S. STERN

Department of Nutrition, University of California, Davis, California

The problem of controlling obesity is one of the most difficult in clinical medicine. Over 30% of the adult women in the United States are diagnosed as obese, which means that they weigh at least 20% in excess of ideal body weight. This prevalence increases with age from 12% for women in their twenties to 46% for women in their fifties (1). Dieting is a national pastime. Of 705 women surveyed, over 45% reported they wanted to lose weight, and 67% admitted that they could not eat whatever they wanted without gaining weight (2).

Treatments for obesity rarely effect a permanent cure, and the majority of individuals that are treated for obesity do not lose any significant amount of weight (3). Even when weight reduction is achieved the recidivism rate is extremely high, with the majority of individuals regaining the lost weight over a period of several years. So called "fad" or "crash" diets designed to take off weight rapidly fail to control obesity because they are not accompanied by a fundamental change in eating habits, except during the relatively short period in which the diet is followed. However, barely a month goes by without the appearance of another revolutionary new diet that promises instant weight loss. Each newly proposed reducing diet continues to excite obese individuals into thinking that somehow the basic laws of conservation of energy are not operative and that by eating a special combination of specific foods or by taking a special pill, they can lose weight with little difficulty, instantly!

Supported in part by NIH grant AM 18899.

Table 1 provides a summary of 15 popular weight control programs. This chapter will analyze several in more depth. Popular strategies can be roughly broken down into the following four areas, which will be considered in order below: drug treatment, dietary treatment, exercise, and group treatment. The effectiveness of any one treatment will be evaluated not only in terms of amount of weight loss but also in terms of dropout rate, length of time of study, composition of weight loss, and health hazards and side effects. For example, many of the often-quoted studies in the weight control literature are short-term studies, some lasting as little as one week. Since obesity, once established, appears to be a lifelong problem, with weight loss often followed by weight regain, the ultimate test of effectiveness of any weight control program should be based on results obtained 1 year, 5 years, or even 10 years later. Few studies of this type are available.

Table 1 15 Diets Rated (Adapted from J. Stern (4))

ANTI-CELLULITE DIET: proposed by Nicole Ronsard, a basically healthful diet, emphasizing raw vegetables, freshly squeezed vegetable juices, lots of water (6–8 glasses per day). You are advised to limit meat, fish, or poultry to broiled, lean cuts.

Cellulite is billed as unevenly distributed lumps of fat caused by, among other things, bad eating habits and not getting enough rest, which ordinary dieting and exercise will not dissolve. Cellulite is no different from ordinary fat . . . it is just fat with a French accent.

DR. ATKINS' REVOLUTIONARY DIET: a variant of the old low-carbohydrate high-protein diet. According to Dr. Robert C. Atkins, weight comes from the body's inability to metabolize carbohydrates properly. He recommends an unlimited consumption of proteins and fats while severely limiting carbohydrates (5).

On this diet, one may lose up to 8 pounds in the first week, but weight loss will be mostly water and as soon as carbohydrates are added to the diet, this lost water is regained. A measure of success is a purple urine-test stick, indicating that your body is in a state of ketosis brought on by a very low carbohydrate diet.

According to The Medical Letter of Drugs and Therapeutics, this diet may result in extreme fatigue, irregular heartbeats, nausea, fainting, calcium depletion. In pregnant women, ketosis may have harmful effects on the unborn child. This high-protein diet is especially harmful to people with undiagnosed kidney disease, and may even precipitate an attack of gout due to high uric acid levels (6).

BANANA-MILK DIET: requiring 6 bananas plus 3 glasses of milk per day, plus vitamin and mineral supplements. Originally developed by Johns Hopkins Hospital (it is also known as the Johns Hopkins Diet) for the use of patients with diabetes, it provides less than 1000 calories per day, has been used for weight reduction, too. As well as being a crashing bore, bananas and milk are not balanced nutritionally. If one tries this diet for more than a few days, be sure to take vitamin and mineral supplements.

CALORIES DON'T COUNT: a low-carbohydrate diet developed by Dr. Herman Taller in the early 1960s. Dr. Taller claims that if you eat the "right" amount of polyunsaturated fat, in the form of safflower capsules and margarine, this stimulates the pituitary gland and gets the body fat burned at a higher rate. The only proven effect of the safflower oil is to add calories—124 per tablespoon. This diet is low in calcium and riboflavin, and could be low in vitamin C if vegetables are not carefully selected.

DRINKING MAN'S DIET: limiting carbohydrates to 60 g/day and allowing you to have filet mignon with sauce Bearnaise and a bottle of your favorite wine, followed by brandy after your espresso. Sounds great—but the same problems apply as with all low-carbohydrate, high-protein diets. Plus, by substituting alcohol for food, you limit your dietary choices and almost ensure that you will not get a well-balanced diet.

THE ICE-CREAM DIET: developed by Gaynor Maddox, a varied, nutritionally well-balanced diet that includes 2 servings of ice cream in its 1000 calories per day plan. If you cannot bear life without ice cream, remember there are only 145 calories in $\frac{1}{2}$ cup of peach Melba parfait ice cream.

LECITHIN, B_6, APPLE-CIDER VINEGAR, AND KELP DIET: Mary Ann Crenshaw's low-calorie diet calls for lecithin (2 tablespoons/day) to help—she claims—emulsify your fat, B_6 to help metabolize your fat, apple-cider vinegar (1 teaspoon after each meal) for potassium and because vinegar and fat do not mix, and kelp (6 tablets after each meal) for iodine to make your thyroid gland speed up your metabolism. In a recent study, Joan Dobbs, a researcher at the University of California at Davis, found that this plan did not speed up weight loss (7).

MACROBIOTICS: a system of diets relying primarily on whole-grain cereal, fish, and selected vegetables. The ultimate diet, according to the late George Ohsawa, Regimen #7 consists of 100% brown rice. Although proponents of macrobiotics claim cures for such diverse maladies as air-sickness and varicose veins, strict adherence to brown rice will result in a lack of such nutrients as protein, calcium, and vitamins A, D, and C, and may even produce signs of frank nutritional deficiencies such as scurvy.

THE MAGIC MAYO DIET (sometimes, the Grapefruit Diet): neither magic nor endorsed by the famous Mayo Clinic, this diet recommends half a grapefruit or grapefruit juice with every meal, all the meat, fish, and eggs you can eat, and limits sugars and starches. The grapefruit is claimed to be "essential" to success, acting as a catalyst that activates fat burning. Not so. While grapefruit is a good source of vitamin C, it is not a mysterious fat catalyst. This diet is high in saturated fats and cholesterol and may be dangerously low in carbohydrates.

SIMEONS HCG (HUMAN CHORIONIC GONADOTROPIN) DIET PLAN: based on daily injections of HCG, a compound obtained from pregnant women's urine, plus adherence to a 500-calorie per day diet. The late Dr. A. T. W. Simeons also restricted the use of cosmetics with oils, since he believed that applied oils can be absorbed and added to your fat stores.

According to Dr. Jules Hirsch and Dr. Theodore Van Itallie, it is probably adherence to the 500 calories, not the HCG injections, that should be credited with the weight loss (8). The AMA has warned against the injections—and we warn against staying on a 500-calorie diet for more than a few days at a time.

ANY STARVATION DIET: simple—just do not eat or drink anything except water and lose 1 pound a day. Some starvation diets permit fruit juices. Proponents of fasting for weight control and spiritual health claim that fasting can help eliminate poisons from the body. Fasting when closely supervised by a physician can be a useful technique for the patient who is morbidly obese. However, one should not go on a starvation diet without close supervision by a physician because of hazards which include ketosis, dehydration, nausea, dizziness, fatigue, and loss of minerals such as potassium, calcium, and magnesium. Another disadvantage: a lot of weight loss is due to loss of muscle and quickly replaced water.

DR. STILLMAN'S QUICK INCHES-OFF DIET: a high-carbohydrate, low-protein diet that forbids meats, seafood, poultry, milk, and cheeses. Dr. Irwin M. Stillman claimed that if one follows this diet one can lose pounds wherever wanted (i.e., spot reduce). According to the U.S. Department of Health, Education, and Welfare, if you have abnormal fat depots and you lose weight, these fat depots will be smaller but still disproportionately large.

DR. STILLMAN'S QUICK WEIGHT-LOSS DIET: high in protein, low in carbohydrate. You do not count calories, and Dr. Stillman lets you eat as much as you want of eggs, meat, poultry, fish, and seafood. You must drink 8 glasses of water each day. Dairy foods, with the exception of cottage cheese, are forbidden. The same cautions apply as for all low-carbohydrate, high-protein diets.

VEGETARIAN DIETS: potentially safe to lose weight. If you will not eat cheese and eggs, be careful to choose foods with high quality protein such as soybeans, and foods with complementary proteins such as beans and rice. Vegetarian diets are high in fiber, can be low in cholesterol (if you limit the number of eggs), and tend to cost less than diets with meat.

WEIGHT-WATCHER'S DIET PLAN: developed by Jean Nidetch and improved by Dr. William H. Sebrell, a noted nutritionist-physician. Nutritionally sound, it has three basic programs—reducing, leveling, and maintenance. You choose from lists of foods, e.g., you are allowed unlimited amounts of "legal" vegetables, such as lettuce, but only moderate amounts of others, such as green beans. It is not the plan for everyone—no one diet is. As with The Diet Workshop and TOPS, equally sound weight-loss plans, the weekly meetings are often quite supportive, but the quality of the meetings greatly depends on the group leader.

DRUG TREATMENT

Most reports involving drug treatment of obesity are relatively short-term studies of several weeks in duration. In a double-blind design, they compare a group receiving a placebo with a group receiving amphetamines or fenfluramine or some other anorexigent agent. There are numerous reports that confirm the effectiveness of these agents in decreasing food intake in the short-term in humans and laboratory animals (9–11). It is not the intent of this chapter to provide an extensive review of the drug treatment literature but merely to provide a framework to evaluate work of this nature. The report of Stunkard and colleagues is illustrative in that it was one of the first studies to compare the relative effectiveness of fenfluramine with an amphetamine (dexamphetamine) (12). Ninety obese women were studied for a period of seven weeks. Body weights were not reported, but the mean percentage overweight was 34%. Patients were randomly assigned to three groups which included a placebo group and the two drug treatment groups. Physicians told their patients that "the capsules supplied might contain a new appetite suppressant which should help them lose weight if they took it regularly for seven weeks." No specific diet was provided but general advice on eating habits was given. Results of this study are given in Table 2. Depending on the

Table 2 Weight Loss during Drug Treatment Program[a]

	Start	3 weeks		5 weeks		7 weeks	
Medication	Number of Patients	Number of Patients	Weight Loss (lb)	Number of Patients	Weight Loss (lb)	Number of Patients	Weight Loss (lb)
Fenfluramine	30	27	4.2	24	4.6	16	6.6
Dexamphetamine	30	27	4.0	21	5.2	15	6.2
Placebo	30	27	0.7	11	4.3	11	5.3

[a] From Stunkard, A., Rickels, K. and Hesbacker, P. (7).

time period examined one could come to different conclusions about the "effectiveness" of the different treatments. If the study had been terminated at 3 weeks, one would conclude while there were no apparent differences between the two drugs, each group losing approximately 4 lb, the placebo was noticeably ineffective in promoting weight loss, with an average of 0.7 lb lost. Although most side effects were relatively mild, side effects were reported by 89% of fenfluramine patients, 44% of dexamphetamine patients and in a surprising 37% of placebo patients. The number of patients reporting side effects decreased with time, presumably because patients experiencing these side effects discontinued the study. If the study had been terminated at 5 weeks, there would appear to be little practical difference between the amount of weight lost in the placebo group (4.3 lb) compared to fenfluramine

(4.6 lb) and dexamphetamine (5.2 lb). In fact the amount of weight loss in the placebo group was greater between the third and fifth week than in the drug treatment groups. However, note the high dropout rate of the placebo group—only 11 of the original 30 patients remained in treatment compared to 21 and 24 patients in the two drug treatment groups. One must assume that the patients that dropped out did so because they did not lose weight; however, these data are not provided. The study was actually terminated at 7 weeks, at which point there were no striking differences in amount of weight loss in any of the groups. Dropout rate was slightly higher in the placebo group but even in the fenfluramine group 14 of the 30 patients did not complete the study and presumably did not lose any weight. Stunkard and his colleagues conclude that despite the limitations of the study "fenfluramine is clearly an effective agent in the treatment of obesity." We question this conclusion in view of the findings that fenfluramine resulted in a weight loss of only 0.9 lb/week compared to 0.7 lb/week in the placebo group. This combined with the high frequency of side effects in the fenfluramine group make it a less than desirable treatment.

Drugs are used not only to suppress appetite but supposedly to help break down fat. There are numerous weight control clinics that utilize a program developed by Dr. A. Simeons which is based on patients' receiving daily injections of human chorionic gonadotropin (HCG), a compound found in pregnant women's urine and following a strict 500 kcal/day diet (13). Patients are instructed to avoid using cosmetics with oils or fats because Dr. Simeons felt that the oils might be absorbed through the skin, possibly hindering weight loss. (Rubbish!) Adherance to the low-calorie, low-fat diet in combination with HCG injections was thought to promote weight loss by inducing lipolysis. There is little evidence that HCG alone promotes lipolysis in adult human adipose tissue (14). However, Asher and Harper in a clinical double-blind trial tested the effects of HCG and dietary restriction on weight loss (15). Forty obese women (20/group) received a daily injection (six per week) of either 125 IU of HCG or saline for six weeks. They were also placed on a low-fat diet of approximately 500 kcal/day. Results are given in Table 3. Note that patients receiving HCG lost significantly more weight than patients receiving saline (20 vs. 11 lb, respectively, $p<.05$). Based on these data as reported by Asher and Harper it appeared that HCG was indeed effective in promoting weight loss. Hirsch and Van Itallie, in a letter to the editor of the *American Journal of Clinical Nutrition*, noted that HCG patients received an average of four more injections than did saline controls (Table 3) (8). They then correlated the number of injections with percent weight loss and reported an r value of $+0.683$ ($p<.05$). The more injections a patient received the more weight she lost. Hirsch and Van Itallie concluded that based on the study of Asher and Harper, individuals that receive more injections may

Table 3 Effect of Administration of Human Chorionic Gonadotropin (HCG) on Weight Loss

Treatment Groups	Number of Injections	Initial Weight (lb)	Weight Loss (lb)	Weight Loss (%)
HCG (n = 20)	33.85 ± 0.85^b	171.71 ± 9.46	19.96 ± 1.63^b	11.47 ± 0.58^b
Placebo	29.05 ± 2.30	164.98 ± 5.78	11.05 ± 1.29	6.77 ± 0.83

[a] Data from Asher, W. L., and Harper, H. W. (15). Results represent mean ± standard error of the mean.
[b] Significantly different from control at $p < .05$.

adhere better to a low-calories diet than those that receive fewer injections. The composition of the injection may make little difference. Certainly it was not possible to come to any conclusion about the efficacy of HCG in weight loss.

While it is possible that in the future successful treatment of obesity may involve some form of drug treatment, it is clear that none of the drugs currently available meets this need.

DIETARY TREATMENT

Numerous studies in the medical literature and at least an equal number of popular diets claim that a particular dietary mixture has a major effect on rate of weight loss. Pennington and Kekwick and Pawan have separately stated that individuals on isocaloric low-carbohydrate, high-protein diets will lose weight more rapidly than individuals on isocaloric high-carbohydrate diets (16, 17). The lay public is more familiar with the best-selling diet books of Dr. I. Stillman (over 5 million copies sold) and Dr. Robert Atkins, which are just variations of this old theme that "calories don't count" (5, 18). All of these studies imply that high-protein diets because of either increased specific dynamic action (SDA) or increased urinary excretion of metabolites such as ketone bodies can account for these remarkable differences in weight loss. These findings are substantiated in the short term (i.e., one to two weeks) but the interpretation over the long term is not valid. Yang and Van Itallie, in a carefully designed study that measured composition of weight loss, demonstrated that the amount of body fat lost was identical for individuals on ketogenic low-carbohydrate diets to the amount of body fat lost by individuals on isocaloric mixed diets that were high in carbohydrate (see Fig. 1) (19). The threefold difference in absolute weight lost in the 10-day period was just

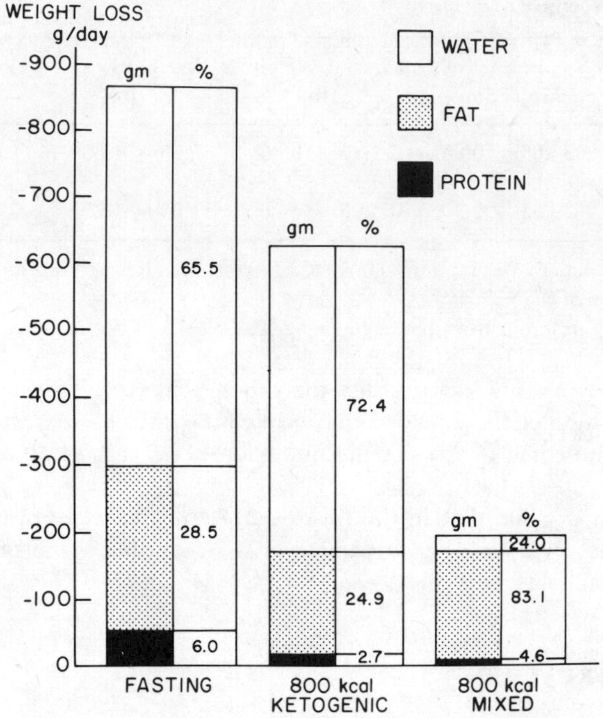

Figure 1. Composition of weight loss during a 10-day period by patients fasting or consuming either an 800 kcal/day ketogenic diet or an 800 kcal mixed diet. M. Yang and T. Van Itallie (19).

due to increased water lost by individuals on the low-carbohydrate diet, which will be predictably regained as soon as carbohydrate is added back to the diet.

Furthermore there is no scientific evidence to indicate that ketogenic high-protein diets have any practical metabolic advantage in weight loss. For example, Bradfield and Jourdan reported that in terms of clinical treatment of obesity, there is no advantage in eating a high-protein diet with the hopes of increasing caloric costs of digestion and assimilation (e.g. SDA) in order to reduce the net calorie value of the diet (20). A calorie is a calorie and in order to lose one pound of body fat there must be a caloric deficit of approximately 3500 kcalories.

Additional studies point out the hazards of reducing diets such as the Atkins and Stillman diets which are dangerously low in carbohydrate and high in animal fat (see Table 1) (6, 21, 22). Hazards include fatigue, nausea, calcium depletion, increased serum cholesterol, kidney failure in individuals predisposed to kidney disease, and attacks of gout in individuals predisposed to gout. The often-quoted study of Rickman and colleagues investigated the effects of feeding Dr. Stillman's Quick Weight Loss (QWL) Diet to 12 volunteers (22). Table 4 compares the QWL Diet with the "average" American

Table 4 Comparison of the Stillman Diet and the "Average American Diet"[a]

	Average Daily American Diet	Stillman Diet
Calories	2565	1325
Total fat		
g	115	73
% of total calories	42	50
Protein		
g	100	160
% of total calories	16	48
Carbohydrate		
g	261	7
% of total calories	42	2
Cholesterol, mg	533	1215

[a] From Rickman, F., Mitchell, N., Dingman, J., and Dalen, J. E. (21).

diet. Note that the QWL Diet provided only 2% of calories (i.e., 7 g) as carbohydrate, along with over 1200 mg of cholesterol. This study lasted approximately 8½ days, during which time the 8 subjects lost approximately 7 pounds, which were 5 pounds more than a predicted weight loss of approximately 2 pounds. Side effects included an increase in serum cholesterol in all subjects from 215 mg/100 ml to 248 mg/100 ml. In addition most subjects complained of fatigue and nausea and several felt that the symptoms interfered with job performance. Within one week after subjects discontinued the diet there was an average weight regain of 4½ pounds (Table 5). Based on the aforementioned study of Yang and Van Itallie these rapid shifts in weight were probably due to loss and regain of body water.

Table 5 Characteristics of Subjects while on the Stillman Diet[a]

Daily caloric intake	1325	Weight loss	6.9 lbs.
Duration	8.4 days	Predicted weight loss	1.8 lbs.
Initial weight	137 lbs.	Weight regain	4.5 lbs.

[a] Data from Rickman, F., Mitchell, N., Dingman, J., and Dalen, J. E. (21).

Long-term studies such as those done by Kinsell and co-workers, where diet composition was changed at three week intervals but weight reduction was measured under controlled conditions for more than two months, provide some of the best arguments against these so-called quick loss diets (23). Despite some day to day variability and some initial water retention when patients are switched from low- to high-carbohydrate diets, weight reduction proceeded in a predictable steady fashion based on caloric intake, independent of composition of the diet. Long-term studies in laboratory animals also support the contention that a calorie is a calorie (24). Low-carbohydrate diets, as expected, have no advantage as reducing diets for rats as compared to other diets on an equal calorie basis (24). Other factors in humans, such as frequency of feeding, do not appear to influence the amount of weight lost over a given time (25, 26).

EXERCISE TREATMENT

Physical activity can be an important factor in determining caloric needs of an individual. Passmore and Durnin reported that a relatively sedentary man (clerk) required approximately 2600 kcal/day to maintain his body weight of 66 kg compared to approximately 4000 kcal/day required by a very active man (coal miner) to maintain his body weight (67 kg) (27). Inactivity may actually promote obesity. Greene, for example, has reported that increased weight gain in 67.5% of adult patients that he studied occurred simultaneously with a decrease in activity (28). Mayer and colleagues studied an industrial population of West Bengal that had a wide range of physical activity (29). Less active individuals ate more and weighed more than active individuals (Fig. 2). This picture is similar to that found in experimental animals where inactivity promotes fattening (30, 31).

Most obese humans are observed to be less active than normal weight individuals (31–33). Not only do they spend less daily time in physical activity, but when actually participating in a given activity, more time is spent at rest. For example, at summer camp obese adolescent girls spend more time compared to lean girls being inactive while participating in scheduled sports programs such as swimming, volleyball, and tennis (Fig. 3, (34)).

While exercise can be an important factor in any weight reduction program, the use of exercise in the treatment of obesity is surrounded by faddism. Reducing salons and magazine advertisements have often promoted the idea that by use of certain vibrating machines one can actually "spot" reduce by mobilizing fat. There is no scientific evidence to support this concept. Gwinup and co-workers measured the thickness of subcutaneous fat at specific sites over the right and left arms of tennis players (36). They found no differences

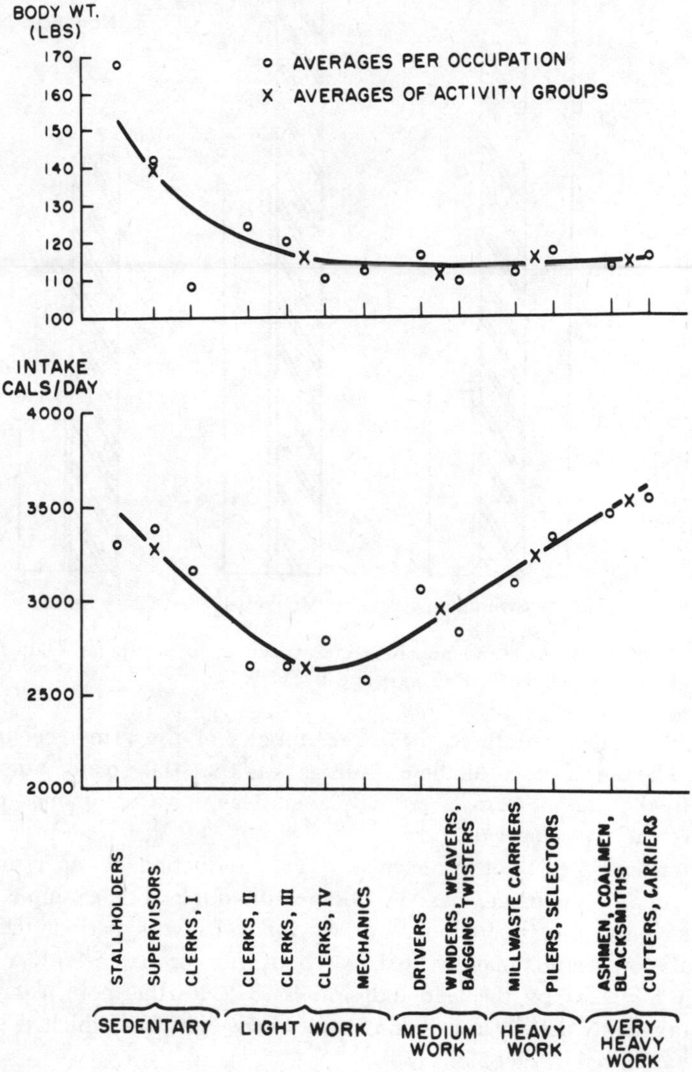

Figure 2. Body weight and caloric intake as a function of physical activity. J. Mayer et al. (29).

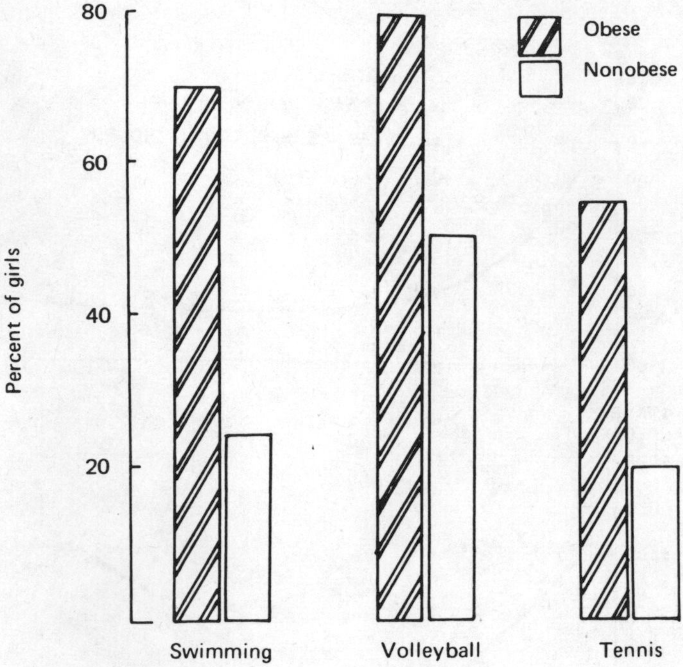

Figure 3. Percent of obese and nonobese girls inactive during sports. Data from B. Bullen et al. (34) as adapted by R. Stuart and B. Davis (35).

in skinfold thickness at three sites over muscles of the arm receiving less exercise. The significance of these findings was that the greater amount of exercise in the playing arm of tennis players was not accompanied by any decrease in fat depots over that arm.

Although exercise is not effective in "spot" reduction, it can result in a decrease in adipose tissue mass in obese individuals. For example, when sedentary young men exercised regularly for a 10-week period, the obese individuals lost approximately 4.8 kg of body fat compared with a loss of 1.8 kg of body fat by the lean individuals (37). Furthermore, exercise in combination with dietary restriction results in weight loss which is greater than that achieved by diet alone (38).

GROUP TREATMENT

A number of successful weight reduction organizations administer their programs in a group setting. In general, the cost to the individual is modest and less than standard medical treatment programs. The question remains is group treatment more or less effective than the standard medical treatment?

London and Schrieber evaluated the effectiveness of group discussions and an appetite suppressant on weight loss over a six-month period (39). They included in their study the first 240 patients admitted to the weight control clinic of an army hospital. Patients were at least 20% above their ideal body weight. All were encouraged to exercise and follow a prescribed diet. There were six regimens including drug treatment (d-amphetamine sulfate-prochlorperazine), placebo, and no medicine, plus these three treatments combined with group discussions (Table 6). Groups met every other

Table 6 Effects of Group Discussions and Drug Treatment on Weight Loss[a]

	Start	6 months	
Regimen	Number of Patients	Number of Patients	Weight lost (lb)
Drug	40	14	10.0 ± 6.6
Placebo	40	19	5.9 ± 3.2
No medicine	40	9	9.8 ± 0.3
Group and drug group	40	32	18.8 ± 5.7
Group and placebo	40	30	14.9 ± 0.9
Group and no medicine	40	25	14.1 ± 2.3

[a] Date from London, A. M., and Schreiber, E. D. (39). Results represent mean values ± standard deviation.

week. Patients not meeting in groups were weighed monthly and were able to consult with the internist or dietitian if they had any questions or problems. At the end of six months of treatment 72.5% of the patients in discussion groups remained in treatment compared with only 35% in the standard medical treatment groups. Of those remaining in the study, patients in group discussions were more successful in losing weight than patients receiving standard medical treatment (16.1 vs 8.1 lbs lost, respectively). There were no significant differences between weight loss of the three group discussion regimens.

Garb and Stunkard evaluated the effectiveness of 21 chapters of TOPS, a 28-year-old self-help organization for the obese (40). Chapters were studied in 1968 and in 1970. Attrition rates were quite high, 47% at one year and 70% at two years. Dropping out was not a measure of success but was associated with smaller weight losses. Mean weight loss was similar in both surveys

(15.0 and 14.2 lbs, respectively). However, there was a large variability in weight loss from chapter to chapter (Fig. 4). In the 1968 survey, the percentage of the members losing at least 20 pounds varied from 62.5% to 4.5%. It was not possible to identify what characteristics of certain chapters contributed to their effectiveness or their lack of effectiveness. Once again the long-term results of most obesity treatment programs are not very impressive.

In 1967, R. Stuart published his results using behavior modification in a group setting for weight control (41). The basic principle behind using behavior modification for the treatment of obesity is the assumption that eating is a learned behavior. If an individual is obese, this behavior is maladapted and should be unlearned and appropriate behavior substituted. A

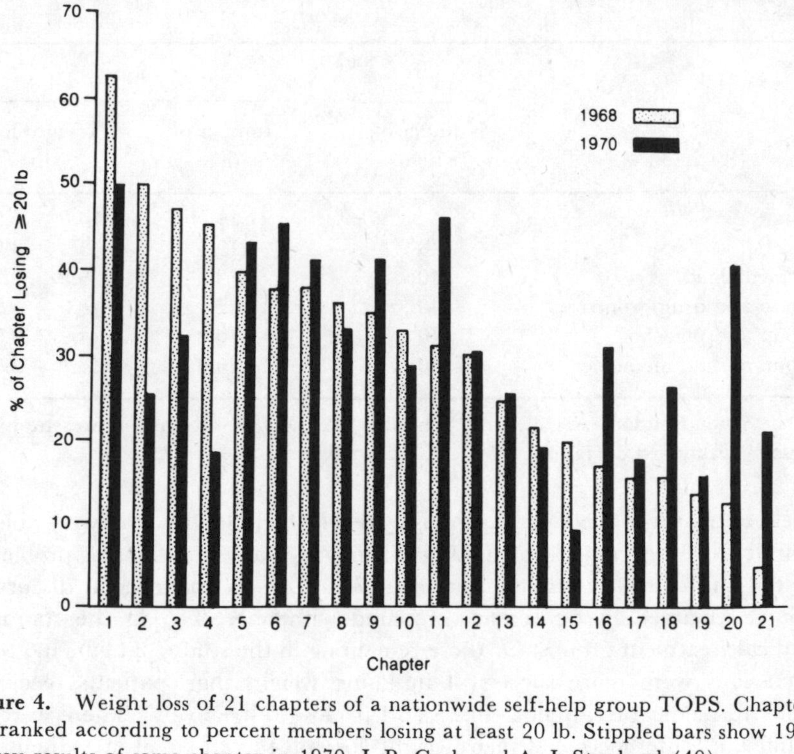

Figure 4. Weight loss of 21 chapters of a nationwide self-help group TOPS. Chapters are ranked according to percent members losing at least 20 lb. Stippled bars show 1968 survey results of same chapter in 1970. J. R. Garb and A. J. Stunkard (40).

step-by-step description of this treatment is given by Stuart and Davis in their book *Slim Chance in a Fat World* (35). Stuart in his original study treated 10 patients for a period of one year (41). Of the 8 patients remaining in the study, all lost more than 20 lb and 6 lost more than 30 lb. Levitz and Stunkard designed a study to see if behavior modification would improve the effectiveness of self-help groups. Sixteen TOPS chapters received one of four treatments: behavior modification conducted by professionals, behavior modification conducted by TOPS' leaders, nutrition education, or the standard TOPS program (42). During the three-month treatment program, fewer TOPS members dropped out of the two behavior modification groups than out of the nutritional education and control groups (Fig. 5). Weight losses were greatest in the behavior modification groups run by professionals (Fig. 6). Furthermore, at a nine-month follow-up this difference was even more striking. Only this behavior modification group did not regain the lost weight, although the average weight loss was only $6\frac{1}{2}$ pounds. Thus introduction

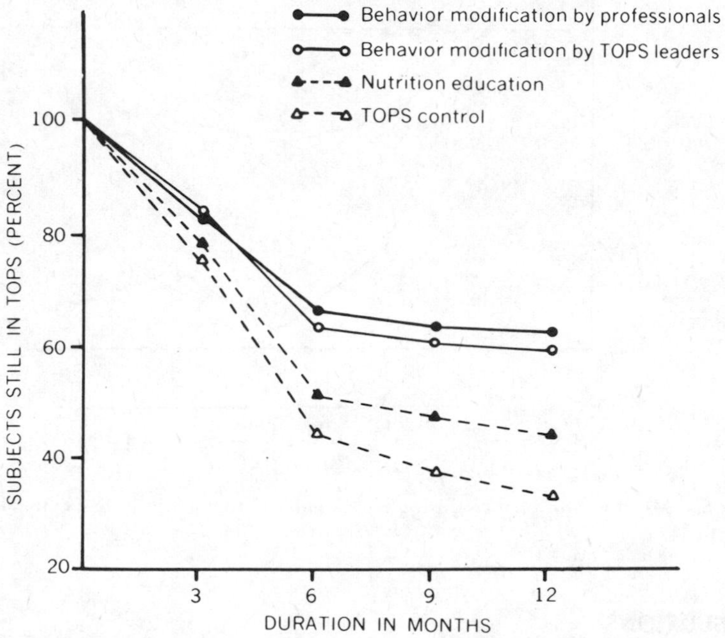

Figure 5. Rates of attrition in four treatment groups. L. S. Levitz and A. J. Stunkard (42).

of behavior modification techniques can improve the effectiveness of self-help groups. Based on this study and several others, behavior modification appears to be more effective in treating obesity than traditional methods. However, longer-term follow-up studies are needed.

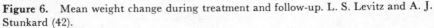

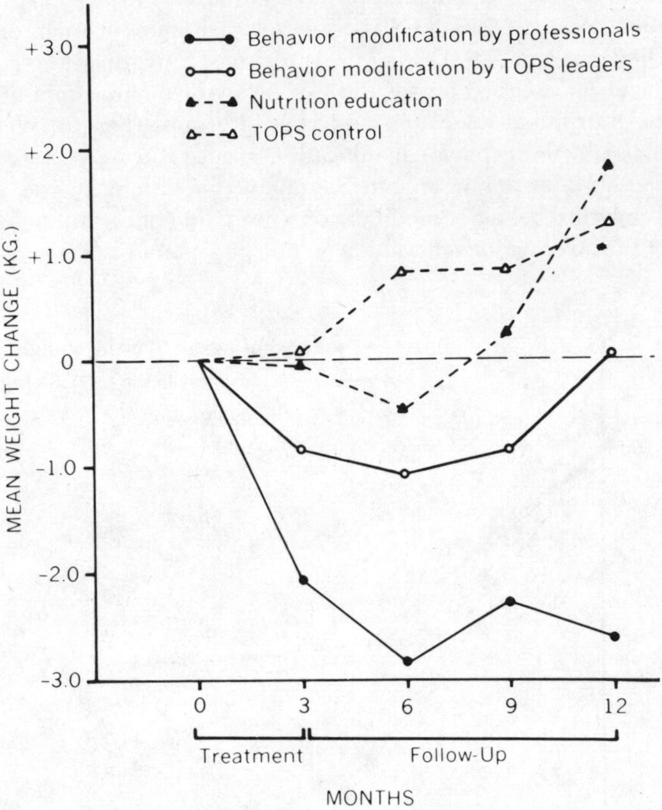

Figure 6. Mean weight change during treatment and follow-up. L. S. Levitz and A. J. Stunkard (42).

CONCLUSIONS

The plethora of treatments for human obesity and their relative ineffectiveness are testimony to the fact that the causes of obesity are still poorly understood. The theories of etiology range from the concept that the obese individual is somehow lazy, has no will power, or just has bad eating habits, all the way to the other side of the spectrum that there is some very esoteric and as yet undiscovered metabolic disorder which leads to increased fate deposition. Until the underlying causes of obesity are elucidated, the successful treatment of this disease will continue to elude us. Yet we are faced with millions of obese individuals who demand some kind of treatment. Based on current knowledge, the most successful weight control programs should include some combination of behavior modification aimed at dietary restriction and an exercise program. For maximum success both should be administered in a group setting.

REFERENCES

1. Metropolitan Life Insurance Co. Frequency of overweight and underweight. *Statistical Bulletin* **41**:4, January 1960.
2. Dwyer, J. T. and Mayer, J. Potential dieters: who are they? *J. Am. Diet. Assoc.* **56**:510 (1970).
3. Stunkard, A. J. and McLaren-Hume, M. The results of treatment of obesity: A review of the literature and report of a series. *Arch. Intern. Med.* **103**:79 (1959).
4. Stern, J. Fifteen diets rated. *Vogue Beauty and Health Guide*, 1975–6, p. 129.
5. Atkins, R. C. *Dr. Atkins Diet Revolution*. McKay, New York, 1972.
6. Anonymous, Dr. Atkins diet revolution. *The Medical Letter on Drugs and Therapeutics* **15**:41 (1973).
7. Dobbs, J., Kime, Z., and Wilmore, J. Manuscript in preparation, 1976.
8. Hirsch, J. and Van Itallie, T. The treatment of obesity. *Am. J. Clin. Nutr.* **26**: 1039 (1973).
9. Booth, D. A. Amphetamine anorexia by direct action on the adrenergic feeding system of the rat hypothalamus. *Nature* **217**:869 (1968).
10. Costa, E. and Gorattini, S., Eds., Amphetamines and related compounds. Proceedings of the Mario Negri Institute for Pharmacological Research, Milan, Italy. Raven, New York, 1970.
11. Hadler, A. J. Studies of aminorex, a new anorexigenic agent. *J. Clin. Pharmacol.* **7**:296 (1967).
12. Stunkard, A., Rickels, K., and Hesbacher, P. Fenfluramine in the treatment of obesity. *Lancet* **1**:503 (1973).
13. Simeons, A. T. W. The action of chorionic gonadotropin in the obese. *Lancet* **2**: 946 (1954).
14. Melichar, V., Razova, M., Dykova, H., and Vizek, K. Effect of human chorionic gonadotropin on blood free fatty acids, glucose and release of free fatty acids from subcutaneous adipose tissue in various groups of newborns and adults. *Biol. Neonate* **27**:80 (1975).
15. Asher, W. L. and Harper, H. W. Effect of human chorionic gonadotropins on weight loss, hunger, and feeling of well-being. *Am. J. Clin. Nutr.* **26**:211 (1973).
16. Pennington, A. W. The use of fat in a weight reducing diet. *Delaware Med. J.* **23**:79 (1951).
17. Kekwick, A. and Pawan, CL.LS. Calorie intake in relation to body weight changes in the obese. *Lancet* **2**:155 (1956).
18. Stillman, I. M. and Baker, S. S. *The Doctor's Quick Weight Loss Diet*. Dell, New York, 1967.
19. Yang, M. and Van Itallie, T. personal communication, 1975.

20. Bradfield, R. B. and Jourdan, M. H. Relative importance of specific dynamic action in weight-reduction. *Lancet* **2**:640 (1973).
21. Rickman, F., Mitchell, N., Dingman, J., and Dalen, J. E. Changes in serum cholesterol during the Stillman Diet. *J.A.M.A.* **228**:54 (1974).
22. Council on Foods and Nutrition. A critique of low-carbohydrate ketogenic weight reduction regimens. A review of Dr. Atkins' diet revolution. *J.A.M.A.* **224**:1415 (1973).
23. Kinsell, L. W., Gunning, G., Michaels, G. P., Richardson, J., Cox, S. E., and Lennon, C. Calories do count. *Metabolism* **13**:195 (1964).
24. Hegsted, D. M., Gallagher, A., and Hanford, H. Reducing diets in rats. *Am. J. Clin. Nutr.* **28**:837 (1975).
25. Gwinup, G., Byron, R. C., Roush, W. H., Kruger, F. A., and Hamwi, G. J. Effect of nibbling versus gorging on serum lipids in man. *Am. J. Clin. Nutr.* **13**: 209 (1963).
26. Young, C. M., Scalan, S. S., Topping, C. M., Simko, V., and Lutwak, L. Frequency of feeding, weight reduction, and body composition. *J. Am. Diet. Assoc.* **59**:466 (1971).
27. Passmore, R. and Drunin, J. Human energy expenditure. *Physiol Rev.* **35**:801 (1955).
28. Greene, J. A. Clinical study of the etiology of obesity. *Ann. Int Med.* **112**:1797 (1939).
29. Mayer, J. Roy, P., and Mitra, K. P. Relation between caloric intake, body weight and physical work: studies in an industrial population in West Bengal. *Am. J. Clin. Nutr.* **4**:169 (1956).
30. Mayer, J., Marshall, N. B., Vitale, J. J., Christensen, J. H., Mashayekhi, M. B., and Stare, F. J. Exercise, food intake and body weight in normal rats and genetically obese adult mice. *Am. J. Physiol.* **177**:544 (1954).
31. Engle, D. J. A simple means of producing obesity in the rat. *Proc. Soc. Exp. Biol. Med.* **72**:604 (1949).
32. Mayer, J. Inactivity as a major factor in adolescent obesity. *Ann. N.Y. Acad. Sci.* **131**:502 (1965).
33. Johnson, M. L., Burke, B. S., and Mayer, J. Relative importance of inactivity and over-eating in the energy balance of obese high school girls. *Am. J. Clin. Nutr.* **37**:4 (1956).
34. Bullen, B. A., Reed, R. B., and Mayer J. Physical activity of obese and nonobese adolescent girls appraised by motion picture sampling. *Am. J. Clin. Nutr.* **14**:211 (1964).
35. Stuart, R. and Davis, B. *Slim Chance in a Fat World*. Research Press, Champaign, Ill., 1972.
36. Gwinup, G., Chelvam, R., and Steinberg, T. Thickness of subcutaneous fat and activity of underlying muscles. *Ann. Intern. Med.* **74**:408 (1971).
37. Buskirk, E. R. Increasing energy expenditure: The role of exercise. In *Obesity*. N. L. Wilson, Ed., Davis, Philadelphia, 1969, p. 163.
38. Buskirk, E. R., Thompson, R. H., Lutwak, L., and Whedon, G. D. Energy balance of obese patients during weight reduction: Influence of diet restriction and exercise. *Ann. N.Y. Acad. Sci.* **110**:918 (1963).

39. London, A. M. and Schreiber, E. D. A controlled study of the effects of group discussions and an anorexiant in out-patient treatment of obesity. *Ann. Intern. Med.* **65**:80 (1966).

40. Garb, J. R. and Stunkard, A. J. Effectiveness of a self-help group in obesity control. *Arch. Intern. Med.* **134**:716 (1974).

41. Stuart, R. Behavioral control of overeating. *Behav. Res. Ther.* **5**:357 (1967).

42. Levitz, L. S. and Stunkard, A. J. A therapeutic coalition for obesity: behavior modification and patient self-help. *Am. J. Psychiatry* **131**:423 (1974).

12

Major Nutrition-Related Risk Factors in American Women

FRANK W. LOWENSTEIN, M.D.

National Center for Health Statistics, Rockville, Maryland

The First Health and Nutrition Examination Survey (HANES) in the United States was conducted between May 1971 and June 1974. It was planned, organized, and executed by the Division of Health Examination Statistics in the National Center for Health Statistics according to a mandate from Congress in the National Health Survey Act of 1956. Three preceeding health surveys had been conducted between 1960 and 1970, but this was the first time a nutrition component had been incorporated to assess and monitor over time the nutritional status of the American people.

A national probability sample of 28,043 persons aged 1 to 74 years was selected in 65 different locations covering the contiguous 48 states. Certain age, sex, and income groups were oversampled, because they are the most vulnerable to nutritional deficiency. They were children aged 1 to 5, women of childbearing age, and older people aged 60 to 74. Furthermore, those groups with an income below the poverty level were oversampled. The half-sample was so designed that it was representative of the total population; it consisted of 14,147 persons of which 10,126 have been examined. The total number of females was 5797, of whom 2750 were between 14 and 44 years of age and 1570 between the ages 45 and 74. Only 258 between the ages of

---

Findings presented are based on the first half of the Health and Nutrition Examination Survey under the Division of Health Examination Statistics, National Center for Health Statistics, Health Resources Administration, U.S. Public Health Service, Rockville, Maryland.

15 and 40 were pregnant, or roughly 5%. The nutrition component of HANES consists of four major parts:

1. Dietary intake based on a 24-hour recall and a food frequency questionnaire.
2. Biochemical levels of various nutrients based on assays of bloods and urine samples.
3. Clinical signs of possible nutrition deficiency disease (as observed by an examining physician).
4. Anthropometric measurements.

Dietary intake and biochemical findings were published in January, 1974 (1). A second report dealing with clinical and anthropometric findings was published in April, 1975 (2).

CLINICAL AND LABORATORY FINDINGS

Iron Deficiency with Anemia

Table 1 presents means, medians, and percentages with low values for hemoglobin and hematocrit in women aged 18 to 44 by income and race. Black women had lower mean values and greater percentages of low values than white women regardless of income. Differences between income groups in the same racial group were less marked for hemoglobin than differences between racial groups. Data on dietary iron intake show low intakes in both racial and income groups, with black women in the below poverty income level group having the lowest intake.

Endemic Goiter

The highest prevalence of grade I goiter, 15.8%, was found in adolescent black girls in the highest income groups; the second highest, 13.4%, in black women aged 18 to 24 in the marginal income group, and the third highest, 12.1%, in white women of the same age and income. The higher prevalence in girls starts at ages 6 to 11, reaches its maximum in young adulthood, and then decreases with age; it remains, however, always greater than that in boys and men. In contrast to grade I goiter, grade II goiter showed the highest prevalence in older women aged 45 to 64.

Calcium-Phosphorus Imbalance

This was diagnosed by means of a positive Chvostek's sign, indicating hyper-

Table 1 Hemoglobin and Hematocrit in Women Aged 18–44 by Income and Race

	Income Below Poverty Level		Income Above Poverty Level	
Biochemical Test	White	Black	White	Black
Hemoglobin g/100 ml				
Mean	13.56	12.68	13.96	13.22
Median	13.65	12.81	14.05	13.22
% with low values	6.84	21.48	4.56	14.09
Hematocrit %				
Mean	40.37	38.38	41.36	40.00
Median	40.84	38.80	41.42	40.44
% with low values	16.34	26.66	10.06	19.72
	Niacin deficiency filiform atrophy			
Age group 45–64				
Male	4.6	5.3	2.7	4.0
Female	1.9	3.3	2.4	5.6
Age group 65–74				
Male	6.0	5.8	2.8	6.9
Female	2.5	3.8	6.7	1.8

irritability of the neuromuscular system as found in tetany due to calcium deficiency. Black adolescent girls in the highest income group showed the greatest prevalence of this sign (20.8%). Even in older women prevalence was still relatively high (11.6% in the 45- to 64-year-old black women in the highest income groups). Prevalence was generally greater in blacks than in whites, regardless of income. Dietary intake data showed median calcium intakes to be generally lower in black girls and women regardless of income. In the 18 to 44 age group, black women reached only 80% or less of the standard.

Niacin Deficiency

Fungiform papillary hypertrophy of the tongue, considered a moderate risk sign, was found more frequently in black adolescent girls and young women (aged 18 to 24) regardless of income than in whites of the same age. Other signs of possible niacin deficiency, however, such as filiform papillary atrophy of the tongue, considered a high risk sign, were more prevalent in older black

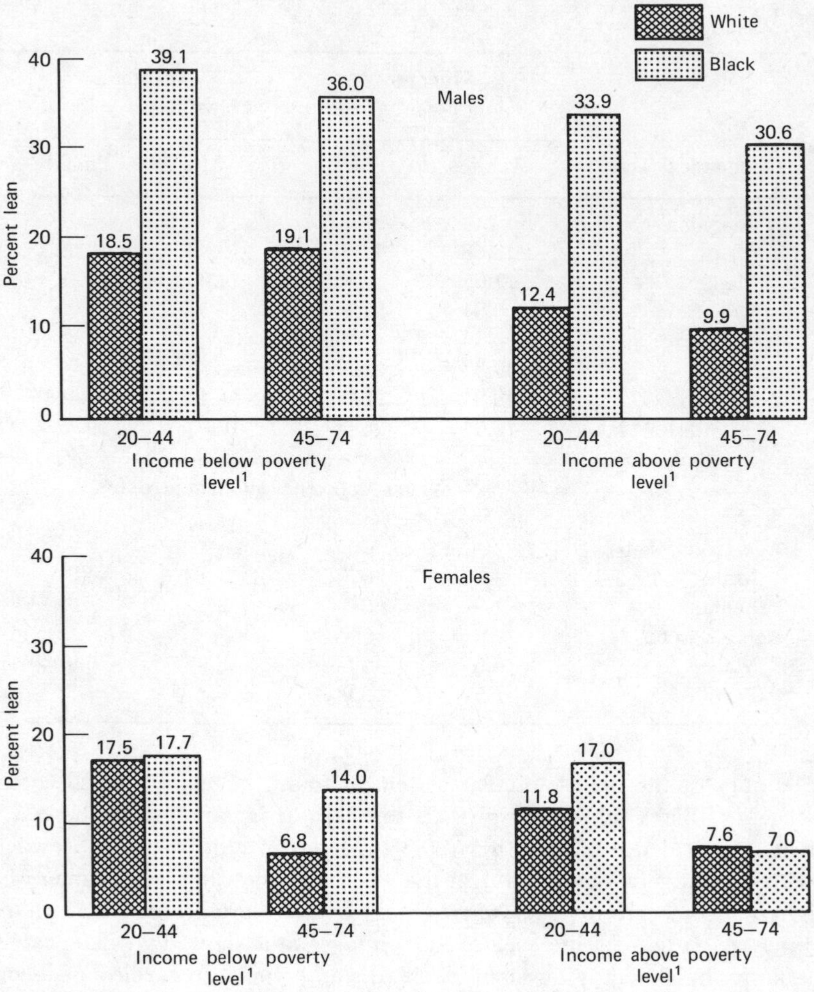

Figure 1. Leanness in American adults, 1971–1972.

males except in two subgroups—black women aged 45 to 64 in the above poverty level income group and white women aged 65 to 74 in the same income group.

ANTHROPOMETRIC FINDINGS

Here data are presented on leanness and obesity in two adult age groups by

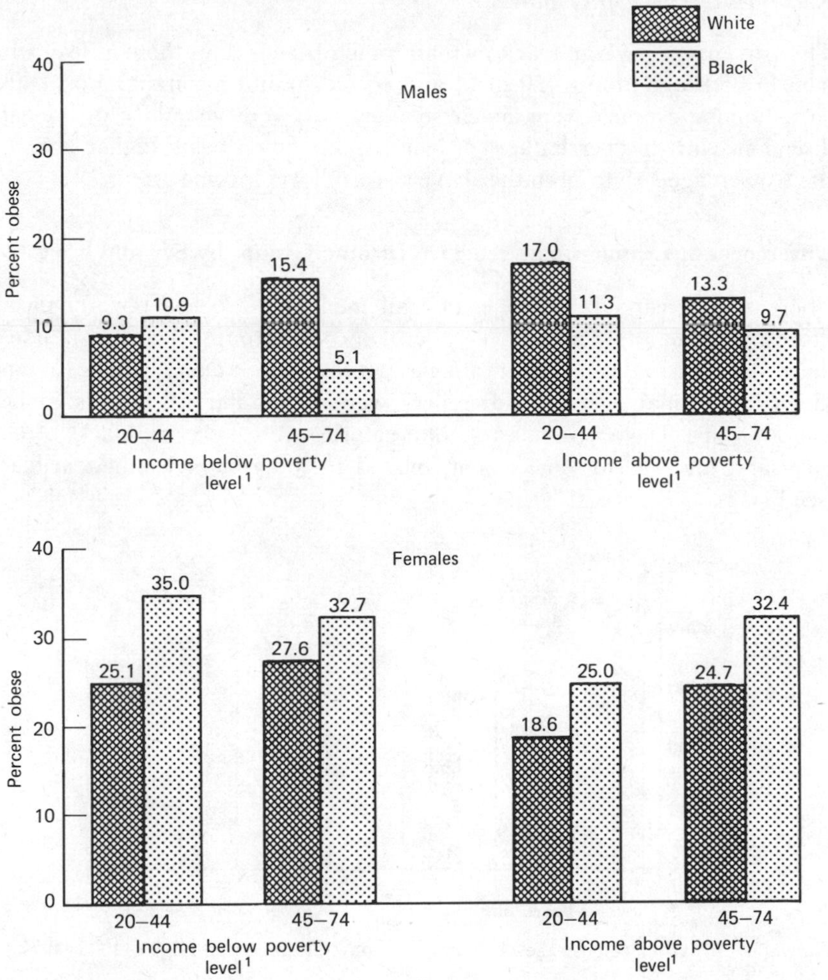

Figure 2. Obesity in American adults, 1971–1972.

race and income. A lean adult was defined as one whose triceps skinfold measurement was less than the sex specific value for the 15th percentile of the distribution of triceps skinfold measurements in the age group 20 to 29 (3). An obese adult was defined as one whose triceps skinfold measurement was more than the sex specific value for the 85th percentile of the distribution of triceps skinfold measurements in the 20 to 29 year age group (2). Figures 1 and 2 present the percentages of lean and obese persons by age, sex, race, and income levels in the United States, 1971–1972.

Racial Differences in Leanness

The percentages of lean black men are much higher than those of lean white men in both age groups (20 to 44 and 45 to 75) and income groups. Differences among women were much smaller, but were generally in the same direction, with the percentages of lean black women being higher except in the women aged 45 to 74 in the above poverty level income group.

Differences in Leanness between Two Income Groups by Sex and Race

There were greater percentages of lean men in the below poverty income groups than in the above poverty level income groups. The magnitude of these differences was greater among whites than among blacks. Women showed a similar picture; differences were of similar magnitude in both racial groups. Dietary intakes of total calories were lower in blacks of both sexes and may be, to some extent, related to the greater leanness in blacks (see Fig. 3).

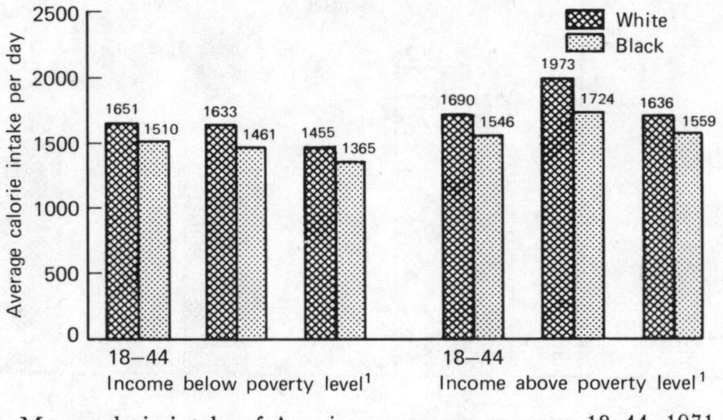

Figure 3. Mean caloric intake of American women, age group 18–44, 1971–1972.

Racial Differences in Obesity

The prevalence of obesity was generally lower among black men than among white men, with the exception of the age group 20 to 44 at below poverty level income. The prevalence of obesity in black women, however, was generally higher than in white women in both age and income groups. Women of all ages had markedly greater percentages of obese than men regardless of race or income. The highest prevalence was reached by black women aged 20 to 44 in the below poverty level income group (35%); in none of the black women's subgroups was the prevalence less than 25%.

Differences in Obesity between Income Groups

The prevalence of obesity in men in the above poverty level income groups was greater than in the below poverty level income groups, except for white men aged 45 to 74. In contrast, women in the below poverty level income groups showed higher percentages of obese at all ages and regardless of race. Caloric intakes (see Fig. 3) were in a different direction, contrary to what might be expected.

DISCUSSION

The prevalence of clinical signs suggesting possible nutrient deficiencies, particularly high risk signs, was generally low. This confirms similar findings from previous surveys such as the Ten-State Nutrition Survey (4) and the Preschool Nutrition Survey (5), which are comparable in many aspects. One can generalize in saying that this situation is probably characteristic for most highly industrialized countries in North America and Europe. Even though dietary inadequacies may be widespread, as in the case of iron, and biochemical tests may show a fairly high percentage of low values, these are usually not severe enough to lead to clinical deficiencies with anatomical lesions in a large number of people. What we are dealing with in a majority of cases is a latent deficiency, which has often been called "subclinical" deficiency, Because of the lack of any true cross correlations at this time between clinical signs on the one hand and biochemical, dietary, and anthropometric findings on the other hand, any interpretation of the above findings must be cosidered tentative and largely speculative. A few observations, however, may be in order. Iron deficiency with anemia has been known to be a public health problem in this country for some time. Our findings in women of childbearing age confirm results obtained in other surveys like the Ten-State Survey (4). This problem is preventable and the means to prevent it are known, but a discussion of this somewhat controversial subject is not within the scope of this chapter.

With the prevalence of endemic goiter above 10% in adolescent black girls and both white and black young women, it presents a public health problem. In a study of adolescents in four states (6), prevalence was also above 10% in girls aged 14 and 16; however, it was not greater in blacks—as in the HANES sample—than in whites. This highest prevalence in adolescent girls corresponds to their known greater susceptibility to thyroid enlargement at that age, Preliminary data on urinary iodine excretion show no relation to goiter prevalence.

Calcium-phosphorus imbalance is usually not mentioned in nutrition surveys although dietary calcium is always looked at and serum levels of calcium and phosphorus are sometimes included. There is suspicion that in highly developed countries calcium-phosphorus imbalance due to relatively lower intake of calcium and higher intake of phosphorus may be a problem. Chvostek's sign is relatively easy to solicit and, if present, indicates increased neuromuscular irritability possibly associated with a relative calcium deficiency. Prevalence of this sign was generally higher in blacks of all ages regardless of income. Prevalence also showed an increase with age over the whole growing period, reaching a peak in adolescent black girls below the poverty income level. Young adults already had a lower prevalence and in the elderly prevalence was as low as in the youngest children. Looking at mean daily calcium intakes per 1000 calories (relative intake), one sees a definite decrease over the whole growing period from age 1 to age 18, which ranges from 57 mg to 134 mg per day in the four subgroups. This decrease in relative calcium intake may be especially critical during puberty, when requirements are increased because of the growth spurt and the final stages of bone growth. A further decrease in relative calcium intake occurs in young adults, which may again be critical for women during pregnancy and lactation. The importance of these findings will be more definitely assessed after data on phosphorus intake and the calcium/phosphorus ratio become available.

Why possible deficiency is more frequent in blacks in general and particularly in adolescents and young women is not known at this time. When dietary intake data become available, cross correlations between niacin intake and clinical signs in some of the subgroups may reveal that one of the causes is dietary deficiency.

In terms of mortality and morbidity greater leanness is an advantage and needs no further discussion in this context. Differences between women by racial and income groups may be explained, to some extent, by similar differences in caloric intake. Obesity, however, shows a different picture: it is inversely related to caloric intake in women. The percentages of black women with obesity are greater than of white women with obesity in all age groups, but black women have lower caloric intakes than white women. There is a negative correlation between total calories and skinfolds and between skinfolds and physical activity. Careful studies in the United States (7) and Great Britain (8) have shown that the obese person may actually eat less than the lean person of the same age, sex, and socioeconomic background, but that the obese moves less and more slowly, thus expending less energy. If the obese person maintains his weight or gains even more weight, it is because he still eats more than he requires. Income is also inversely related to obesity in women of all ages. This occurs only in North America and Western Europe and is probably socioculturally determined. This influence of socioeconomic and cultural factors in obesity has been clearly shown by Goldblatt and coworkers (9) in New York City.

What are other causes of greater obesity in black women? Why do they seem to gain weight more rapidly and easily than whites? What are the differences in body composition if any? The one thing that is known is that blacks have heavier bones than whites and other racial groups (10). In rural Yoruba in Western Nigeria, Edozien (11) found a greater extracellular fluid space and a probably greater muscle mass than in urban educated Yoruba. What is the significance of these differences and do similar differences exist in North America and the Caribbean? Our ignorance is obvious, but these questions must be studied and answered because they have practical importance in setting the standards used in assessing obesity. In the United States, we use the same weight standards for blacks as for whites and other racial groups. These standards are based on life insurance data in Caucasians. They may not apply to blacks and others if real differences in body composition exist. One-third of all black women are obese and stay obese regardless of income. They pay a high price in terms of morbidity and mortality from chronic degenerative diseases associated with obesity, such as hypertension, diabetes, gallbladder disease, heart disease, and osteoarthritis.

The association of obesity and hypertension may be explained through such hemodynamic mechanisms as increased cardiac output, increased blood volume and plasma volume, and such hormonal imbalances as increased adrenocortical function and imbalance of the renin-angiotensin-aldosterone system (12). In the Framingham study (13) an increase of 1:7 in the morbidity ratio between normal weight and obese persons for hypertension was observed and of 1:10 for hypertensive heart disease. Obese hypertensive persons experience a greater risk of coronary heart disease and mortality than persons with either hypertension or obesity alone. The longevity of women at corresponding degrees of overweight and hypertension is much less affected than that of men. With a reduction in weight, the blood pressure usually falls. This risk factor is amenable to correction through reduced caloric intake, low sodium intake, and a cautious exercise program. The association between obesity and diabetes is well documented (14, 15). Eighty per cent of the maturity-onset diabetes occurs in obese individuals; on the other side of the coin, 60 to 70% of grossly obese adults are diabetic or potential diabetics. Diabetes in the obese causes more than three times the expected mortality (16). Black women showed a definite increase of both systolic and diastolic blood pressure with increasing blood glucose levels after age 35 (17). The obese and the maturity-onset diabetic have metabolic defects in common, such as reduced glucose oxidation and hyperinsulinism (18). Weight reduction in the obese diabetic improves glucose tolerance and normalizes serum insulin levels. The association between obesity and heart disease is due, in part, to the effect of an increased workload on the heart. This applies to various types of heart disease, such as hypertensive, arteriosclerotic, and coronary heart disease. Definitive and suspected hypertensive heart disease was between two and five times more prevalent in black women at all ages than in white women in the United States in 1960–1962 (19). Definite and suspected coronary heart disease generally also showed a higher prevalence in black women (19). However, that this may not be true everywhere was shown in the Evans County study (20), where coronary heart disease rates were similar in black and white women at lower levels of risk factors, but at higher levels white women had higher rates. Mean cholesterol levels were lower in older black women aged 45 to 74 in Evans County than in the national sample. Mortality from hypertension (21), diabetes (22), and heart disease (19) is higher in black women than in white women of the same age and socioeconomic level.

Gallbladder disease, according to medical history information in a large sample of women enrolled in a TOPS weight control program (23), was increased with increasing obesity and parity in the younger women (aged 20 to 39).

Mild and severe osteoarthritis was more prevalent in black women aged 25 to 54 in urban areas than in white women (24). Correlation between weight, right arm girth, and triceps skinfolds on the one hand and osteoarthritis of the hands on the other was highly significant in women aged 45 to 54 ($p > .0005$) (25).

SUMMARY AND CONCLUSIONS

Results based on preliminary findings from the Health and Nutrition Examination Survey in 1971–1972 have been presented for women in the United States. From the clinical and laboratory findings, iron deficiency with anemia, endemic goiter, possible calcium-phosphorus imbalance, and niacin deficiency appeared to be major problems in American women. Generally, black women were more affected than white women of the same age, sex, and income group. Differences between below poverty level and above poverty income groups seemed to be less important.

Anthropometric measurements provided data on leanness and obesity. Leanness was defined as a triceps skinfold above the 85th percentile of the distribution by sex. There were more lean black women than whites except in the age group 45 to 74 above poverty level income. There were more obese black women regardless of age and income than white women. One-third of all younger black women were found to be obese and stayed obese in later life. Income differences were again of less importance. In terms of risk of suffering and dying from certain chronic diseases associated with obesity, obese black women are the highest risk group. They deserve special attention in both control and preventive programs.

REFERENCES

1. Preliminary Findings of the First Health and Nutrition Examination Survey, United States, 1971–1972: Dietary Intake and Biochemical Findings. PHS, DHEW Publication No. (HRA) 74–1219–1, 1974.
2. Preliminary Findings of the First Health and Nutrition Examination Survey, United States, 1971–1972: Anthropometric and Clinical Findings. PHS, DHEW Publication No. (HRA) 75–1229, 1975.
3. Unpublished data provided by Mr. Sidney Abraham, Chief, Nutrition Statistics Branch, National Center for Health Statistics, Division of Health Examination Statistics, Rockville, Maryland.
4. *Ten-State Nutrition Survey, 1968–1970 III—Clinical.* PHS, DHEW Publication No. (HSM) 728131, Atlanta, Georgia, 30333.
5. Owen, G. M. et al. A Study of Nutritional Status of Preschool Children in the United States, 1968–1970. *Pediatrics* **35**:4 (1974).
6. Trowbridge et al., Iodine and Goiter in Children. *Pediatrics* **50**:1 (1975).
7. Johnston, M. L. et al. Relative Importance of Inactivity and Overeating in the Energy Balance of Obese High School Girls. *Am. J. Clin. Nutr.* **4**:37 (1956).
8. Durnin, J. V. G. A. Age, Physical Activity and Energy Expenditure. *Proc. Nutr. Soc.* **25**:107–113, 1966.
9. Goldblatt, P. B. et al. Social Factors in Obesity. *J.A.M.A.* **192**:12 (1965).
10. Baker, P. T. and Angel, J. L. Old age changes in bone density: Sex and race factors in the United States. *Hum. Bio.* **37**:104 (1965).
11. Edozien, Joseph C. The role of chemical pathology in rural health investigations. *Ghana Med. J.* **4**:1 (1965).
12. Chiang, B. et al. Overweight and Hypertension. *Circulation* **39**:415 (1969).
13. Kannel, W. et al. Adiposity, blood pressure and hypertension. *Am. Int. Med.* **67**:481 (1967).
14. Drash, Allan, Obesity and diabetes in adolescents. *Florida St. Med. J.* **585**:38 (1971).
15. West, Kelley, Epidemiology of Adiposity Regulation of Adipose Tissue Mass. *Excerpta Medica International Congress Series,* No. 315, Proc. 4, International Meeting of Endocrinology, J. Vague and J. Boyer, Eds., 1973.
16. Armstrong, D. et al. Obesity and its relation to health and disease. *J.A.M.A.* **147**: 1007 (1951).
17. Florey, C. and Acheson, R. Blood pressure as it relates to physique, blood glucose and serum cholesterol. NCHS Series 11, No. 34, U.S. Dept. of Health, Education and Welfare, Washington, D.C., 1969.
18. Gordon, Edgar, Obesity: Gluttony or genes? *Postgrad. Med.* **45**:95 (1969).
19. Gordon, T., Heart disease in adults. NCHS Series 11, No. 6, U.S. Dept. of Health, Education, and Welfare, Washington, D.C., 1964.

20. Tyroler, H. A. et al. Coronary heart disease in Evans County, Georgia. *Arch. Int. Med.* **128:**907 (1971).
21. Roberts, J. Blood Pressure of Persons 18–74 Years, United States, 1971–1972. PHS, DHEW Publication No. (HRA) 75-1632, 1975.
22. Garst, C. C. Blood Glucose Levels in Adults, United States—1960–1962. PHS Publication No. 1000, Series 11, No. 18, 1966.
23. Rimm, Alfred A. et al. Relationship of Obesity and Disease in 75,532 Weight Conscious Women. *Public Health Reports* **90:**44 (1975).
24. Roberts, J. and Burch, T. A. Osteoarthritis Prevalence in Adults by Age, Sex, Race, and Geographic Area, United States, 1960–1962. PHS Publication No. 1000, Series 11, No. 15, 1966.
25. Engel, A. Osteoarthritis and Body Measurements. NCHS Series 11, No. 29, U.S. Dept. of Health, Education, and Welfare, Washington, D.C., 1968.

Index